Complementary Medicine

Complementary Medicine

An objective appraisal

Edited by

Professor Edzard Ernst MD PhD
Director
Department of Complementary Medicine
Postgraduate Medical School
University of Exeter
UK

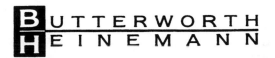

Butterworth-Heinemann
Linacre House, Jordan Hill, Oxford OX2 8DP
A division of Reed Educational and Professional Publishing Ltd

℞ A member of the Reed Elsevier plc group

OXFORD   BOSTON   JOHANNESBURG
MELBOURNE   NEW DELHI   SINGAPORE

First published 1996
Reprinted 1997

British Library Cataloguing in Publication Data
A catalogue record for this book is available from the British Library

Library of Congress Cataloguing in Publication Data
A catalogue record for this book is available from the Library of Congress

ISBN 0 7506 3141 4

Typeset by Keytec Typesetting Ltd, Bridport, Dorset
Printed and bound in Great Britain by
Biddles Ltd, Guildford and King's Lynn

Contents

List of contributors

Anton J. M. de Craen MSc
Department of Clinical Epidemiology and Biostatistics,
Academic Medical Center, Amsterdam, The Netherlands

David P. S. Dickinson MA
Editor, *Health Which?*, Consumers' Association, London, UK

David M. Eisenberg MD
Assistant Professor of Medicine, Harvard Medical School, Boston,
Massachusetts, USA

Edzard Ernst MD PhD
Director, Department of Complementary Medicine, Postgraduate
Medical School, University of Exeter, Exeter, UK

Roger A. Edwards ScD
Instructor in Medicine, Harvard Medical School, Boston,
Massachusetts, USA

Adrian Furnham DPhil DSc DLitt
Professor of Psychology, Department of Psychology, University
College London, London, UK

Wayne B. Jonas MD
Director, Office of Alternative Medicine, United States National
Institutes of Health, Rockville, Maryland, USA

Ted J. Kaptchuk OMD
Instructor in Medicine, Harvard Medical School, Boston,
Massachusetts, USA

Jos Kleijnen MD PhD
Department of Clinical Epidemiology and Biostatistics,
Academic Medical Center, Amsterdam, The Netherlands

George T. Lewith MA DM MRCP MRCGP
Hon. Clinical Senior Lecturer, University Medicine, Southampton
General Hospital, Southampton, UK

Karl-Ludwig Resch MD PhD
Senior Lecturer, Department of Complementary Medicine,
Postgraduate Medical School, University of Exeter, Exeter, UK

Andrew Vickers
Director, Information Service, The Research Council for
Complementary Medicine, London, UK

Adrian R. White MA BM BCh
Research Fellow, Department of Complementary Medicine,
Postgraduate Medical School, University of Exeter, Exeter, UK

Preface

Complementary medicine (CM) has undoubtedly become 'big business'. One third to one half of the general population is using one or more forms of complementary therapy. Sales of herbal and homoeopathic remedies are associated with annual growth rates of around 20%. In addition, more and more institutions are training would-be practitioners. Users of CM are prepared to pay considerable sums out of their own pocket. Also, an increasing number of health insurance companies are willing to take over some of the costs for CM. This growing interest in CM is also reflected in the literature – since 1966 there has been a six-fold increase in the number of CM-related publications in mainstream medical journals.

It is hardly surprising then, that a veritable plethora of books on various aspects of CM is available in our bookshops. One disappointing but outstanding hallmark of this literature is its uncritical nature. Some of these publications are hardly more than promotional texts written by, at best, the well-meaning and read by the gullible. Even some volumes written for professionals and aspiring to an academic standard suffer from being overtly promotional. There are certainly few books available where the author(s) has made a serious attempt to objectively assess CM in general terms and to explore the numerous open questions related to it.

The flurry of interest in CM seems sharply contrasted by an astonishing and embarrassing lack of knowledge in and information on the subject. The void even relates to the most fundamental questions. Does CM work? Is it safe? Can it reduce healthcare costs? How can it be researched?

This volume aims at filling this most obvious gap. It consists of ten contributions by experts from various countries, each of whom looks critically and constructively at a fundamental aspect of CM. The book is neither confined to the agenda of a particular nation, nor does it express the views of either proponents or opponents of CM, nor is it confined to specific therapies, nor is it a book solely written by doctors or by lay-practitioners. It provides balanced and informed views on fundamental, general issues within CM and is aimed at *all* professionals who are seriously interested in the topic.

If the present popularity of CM is to be more than yet another passing fashion, it is essential to cultivate constructive criticism, informed debate and balanced views. Paradoxical as it may seem, those who are inspired by an attitude of constructive criticism will surely turn out to be the true champions of CM, while the naive smugness that is still regrettably prevalent will prove to be counterproductive and, more importantly, against the interests of the patient.

I thank all contributors, the Ciba-Foundation and the publishers for their help in creating this book. I sincerely hope that it will form an important landmark on the way to an understanding of CM that is based more and more on reliable evidence and less and less on personal belief.

Edzard Ernst, Exeter

Chapter 1

Research paradigms in mainstream and complementary medicine

Andrew Vickers

Summary

Our worlds are built up from profound and often hidden assumptions about the nature of reality. These assumptions tend to vary between individuals and groups in systematic ways. Some writers on complementary medicine research have used the term 'paradigm' to capture this idea of conceptual differences between different systems of medicine. I will argue that the notion of a paradigm is not a useful generalization in the methodological debate. Effort seems better spent on the practical matter of how particular research questions can be matched to particular research designs than on esoteric debates about the vague and slippery notion of the paradigm.

Introduction

The concept of the paradigm has become an institutionalized feature of complementary medicine research. Perhaps the best example of this is *The Journal of Alternative and Complementary Medicine*, which describes its aim as 'research on paradigm, practice and policy'. When the Office of Alternative Medicine was established as part of the National Institutes for Health, paradigms even made it to government. The Chantilly report – which outlines the goals of the newly formed office – explicitly states that a major barrier to alternative medicine is that it has a different paradigm to mainstream medicine (National Institutes for Health, 1994).

'Paradigm' is a term borrowed from the history and philosophy of science. It was introduced in 1962 in a text written by Thomas Kuhn, a historian at Princeton University. A year earlier, Nagel had published *The Structure of Science*, a conventional textbook of the philosophy of science: inductive and deductive logic were compared, the problem of the theory laden nature of observations analysed, the difficulty of choosing between two theories – T_1 and T_2 – discussed at length. Kuhn's book had an almost identical title, but the addition of a single word could not have been more significant. In *The Structure of Scientific Revolutions*, Kuhn brought a historian's eye to the philosophy of science. The interesting thing about science, according to Kuhn, was change. Moreover, change did not necessarily happen gradually. Science was not just a steady accumulation of facts, it sometimes involved revolutions in which knowledge was radically reconstituted. Scientific revolutions allowed the incorporation of new facts which failed to fit previous theories ('anomalies') and cast existing knowledge in a new light. Kuhn's most notable example of a scientific revolution was that initiated by Copernicus. The suggestion that the earth orbits the sun goes beyond a mere change in theory: Copernican astronomy involves the replacement of key cosmological concepts such as the immutability of the heavens and the Aristotelian notion that the earth and heavens are subject to different physical laws. Kuhn described such revolutions as a shift from one paradigm – a pattern of seeing the world – to another.

Kuhn's thesis was subjected to bitter attack as soon as it was published. Conservative critics claimed that Kuhn had reduced science to fashion. If all that changed in science were general views about how the world was constituted, and if these views were themselves not testable, how could science be said to progress towards the truth? How could science be said to be rational if important changes – scientific revolutions – did not take place by rational processes? Sympathetic critics pointed out that, though of interest, Kuhn's ideas were often too ambiguous to be of significant explanatory value. The concept of the paradigm was a prime example: Masterman (1965), for example, claimed that Kuhn used the term in 21 different ways.

The argument presented in *The Structure of Scientific Revolutions* is no longer current in the philosophy of science. It is typically taught as a historical introduction, as a background to contemporary debates. What was valuable about Kuhn's theory was the demonstration that change in science can be discontinuous and that scientific theories make relatively global assumptions about both the nature of reality and how to find out about it. Perhaps of greatest importance was Kuhn's insistence that philosophical analysis of science should be rooted in what has happened in the real world: rather than 'T_1' and 'T_2', Kuhn discussed Copernicus, Newton, Preistley and Lavoisier. What was less salutary was the attempt to use large, simple concepts to explain local, complex events. In retrospect it seems naive to suppose that the historical development of a human activity as rich and complex as science can be described in terms of one paradigm replacing another during a scientific revolution. It is also interesting that, despite Kuhn's empirical orientation, the debates about the nature of science following the publication of *The Structure of Scientific Revolutions* (e.g. see

Lakatos and Musgrave, 1965) were almost completely devoid of examinations of what scientists actually did: reference to sociological studies of science and scientists were few and far between.

Given that the concept of paradigms has just about left contemporary discourse in the philosophy of science, it is strange to see it playing such a central role in the debate about complementary medicine research. It is my contention that the notion of the paradigm has been of little practical value in this methodological debate. If anything, it has hindered the development of clear ideas about how complementary medicine should be researched. This is partly because discussion about paradigms seems almost inevitably to involve the use of esoteric and obscure language. But it is also because those writing about paradigms have often articulated the idea crudely and have made over-simplistic assumptions about what they claim to describe. In short, it is difficult to apply big, simple generalizations to complex, real world situations.

The paradigm argument in complementary medicine research

There is no single line of thought common to all of those who write about paradigms in complementary medicine research. However, it is possible to discern a number of themes which are common among those who use the concept of paradigms. The general argument about paradigms has been presented to me orally on numerous occasions at conferences, seminars, lectures and other meetings and it is possible to find important strands of this argument in the methodological literature.

The argument goes as follows: there is such a thing as paradigms; these govern the way we look at the world. There are two entirely separate paradigms, one associated with orthodox medicine and one with complementary medicine. Research methods are paradigm-specific, in other words, research methods used in one paradigm cannot be used in another. Therefore conventional research methodology is inappropriate for complementary medicine. Those working in a paradigm are unable to look outside of it. Conventional scientists are therefore blind to important healing phenomena. Partly because of this, the current medical paradigm is outdated and is about to be replaced. This is a good thing because the methodologies of the orthodox paradigm have had adverse effects on medicine and society and have been nothing less than tools of oppression.

I do not agree with this argument and I will challenge each step in turn.

The concept of a paradigm in complementary medicine research is a meaningful one

One remarkable feature of the current methodological discourse on paradigms is that the term is so rarely explained. 'Paradigm' tends to be used without an accompanying definition or discussion, as though it has an unambiguous and widely understood meaning. Given that researchers often fail to agree on the meaning of terms such as 'audit', 'primary health care' or 'basic research', and given that Kuhn himself used the term in as many as 21 different ways (Masterman, 1965), this assumption is unhelpful at best.

However, when a definition of paradigm is presented, we are often none the better for it. In an explanatory footnote to the Chantilly report (National Institutes for Health, 1994), the Office of Alternative Medicine defines paradigm as an 'overarching cosmological conceptual scheme' which 'tells whole societies in whole historical periods how to think about ... big issues. This is contrasted with an explanatory model, which is 'the way one discipline, denomination or health care system explains itself – the details of its assumptions, logic and rationale'. It is also claimed that whereas a paradigm is largely out of awareness, an explanatory model is not, and is therefore open to argument, criticism and change. Yet in the accompanying text, the first mention of paradigm is followed by the words, 'i.e. broad views of how ... facts should be organized. Differences in views among groups of people are a reflection of the different scientific paradigms they adhere to'. If the groups of people are part of the same society in the same historical period, and if, as it appears, those who hold broad views of how facts should be organized are aware that they are doing so, the definition of 'paradigm' in the text now sounds somewhat like the definition of 'explanatory model' given in the footnote. Consequently, two inconsistent interpretations of 'paradigm' appear on the same page.

The root of this inconsistency is that it is unclear at what metaphysical level paradigms operate. Are paradigms global and all encompassing (whole societies in whole historical periods) or do they refer to 'particular groups of people'? Rubik (1994) talked in the former terms when she spoke of 'the dominant paradigm of mechanical reductionism that shaped science for the past few centuries ... [and] still governs modern biology and medicine'. Coulter (1990) suggested a more localized meaning for the concept of the paradigm when claiming that homoeopathy, osteopathy, naturopathy and chiropractic constituted four separate paradigms in the latter half of the 19th century in North America. Similarly, when Korr (1991) talked of paradigms as 'investigative strategies' and Coulter (1993) discussed the 'alternative social science paradigms', the concept seems to refer to the specific rather than the general.

In sum, the meaning of 'paradigm' remains impenetrable, a feature that could be said to characterize much of the language used in discussions of the concept. Watson (1995) talked of moving from 'a separatist-interactionist ontology to a relational-transformative ontology of connectedness and unity of life itself'. Later she claimed that 'the paradigm I, particular-deterministic model parallels era I medicine described by Dossey as body-machine, mechanical-material physical medicine, and "doing" therapies'. It is hard to see how the use of such obscure language advances either the methodological debate, or our understanding of the differences between medical philosophies.

There is a more fundamental point to be made with respect to paradigms, language and communication. At first sight, the concept of the paradigm seems to be about acknowledging that there are different ways of looking at the world and that we should try to understand each other's points of view. Some methodological writers, however, seem to use the concept to demonstrate the impossibility of discourse. Launsø (1994), for example, stated that complementary medicine 'must produce a knowledge system other than the mechanistic-objectifying paradigm'. Perhaps more worrying, is the statement from the Chantilly report that 'differences in views among groups of people are a reflection of the different scientific paradigms they adhere to'. Given the earlier suggestion that, unlike an explanatory model, a paradigm is not open to argument, the implication of this statement is that people holding different views cannot talk to one another. I hold one view, you hold a different one and there's nothing we can do about it because we have different paradigms. A paradigm can become an 'inference ticket': claiming that you are in a different paradigm gives you a ticket to make whatever inference you please.

A further argument against the concept of paradigm in complementary medicine research is that of *parsimony*. In short, why use a concept if it is not necessary to do so? Many of the arguments around the issue of paradigms would continue to make perfect sense even if the authors did not make reference to the term. For example, Rubik (1994) analysed the obstacles facing scientists working in unusual areas of science ('frontier science') and claimed that these stem from resistance of the dominant paradigm to 'anomalies' (a Kuhnian expression). However, the problems encountered by frontier scientists can be explained on a case-by-case basis without reference to paradigms. The resistance to say, Semmelweiss, is better understood by close historical analysis than by a quick reference to paradigms. It seems more valuable to say that Semmelweiss was scorned by his peers because of his implicit criticism of physicians – and the lack of a theory to account for his observations – than merely to say that he discovered an anomaly which challenged the dominant paradigm. Looking more specifically at research methodology, both Korr (1991) and Masarsky and Weber (1991) provided excellent analyses of research questions pertinent to osteopathy and chiropractic (e.g. is 'upper cervical dysfunction ... more common in (adductor-type spasmodic dysphonia) patients than in the population at large?'). They claimed that these questions stemmed from a paradigm, but it is entirely unclear whether this statement provides any useful additional information. The authors may have been better off stating simply that the questions were suggested by the theory and practice of osteopathy and chiropractic.

There can be little doubt that our worlds are built up from profound and hidden assumptions about the nature of reality. Moreover, these assumptions tend to vary between individuals and groups in systematic ways. As Coulter (1990) put it: 'chiropractors begin with a different set of assumptions, use different theoretical explanations, embrace a different philosophy, pose different questions and use a different language ... than medicine'. But this does not imply that the concept of a paradigm is a useful generalization, or that differences in beliefs and attitudes of individuals and groups cannot be identified and explored on a case-by-case basis. Explicit and implicit assumptions of medical systems need to be teased out and examined individually or in groups. Their implications need to be analysed and discussed and solutions to possible misunderstandings developed. It may be that some aspects of some medical systems cannot be understood as completely in terms used outside of that system, in the same way that *esprit de corps* has an immediate meaning in French which is not easy to describe in English. However, merely asserting that there are profound differences between 'paradigms' seems to take us no further in this project of analysis and understanding. Paradigms might well have a useful conceptual role in some fields of discourse; it has yet to be argued that this is the case in complementary medicine research.

There are two entirely separate paradigms, one associated with orthodox and one with complementary medicine

In a discussion of Chinese medicine, Beinfield and Korngold (1995) included a drawing of two hollow human forms, one labelled West and the other East. Whereas West consisted of mechanical levels and joints and test tubes, the body of East was filled with mountains, clouds, rivers and gardens. This diagram was presented to demonstrate the difference between entirely separate and non-overlapping medical philosophies. In the western biomechanical model, the body is 'like a machine which can be dismantled and reduced into ... constituent parts'; medicine is a 'war on disease with doctor as general, disease as enemy, patient as occupied territory'. In the eastern holographic model, however, the view of anatomy and physiology is that of the 'body as garden' so that the aim of health care is to 'cultivate health with doctor and patient in partnership to improve ecological conditions'.

Beinfield and Korngold presented perhaps the most explicit articulation of the idea that the differences between complementary and conventional medicine are profound – that beyond the superficial distinctions of legal status and treatment techniques lies something more: a clash of world-views, a mismatch of paradigms. Though superficially attractive, and though it does contain a kernel of truth, the notion that complementary and conventional medicine have different paradigms is deeply flawed. This is because it assumes the heterogeneity of medical systems, that complementary medicine is all one thing and conventional medicine is all something different. Such an assumption does scant justice to the range and variety of medical practices. It is not difficult to argue that there can often be greater differences within complementary or conventional medicine (psychotherapy and physical therapy; chiropractic and radionics) as between the two (chiropractic and physical therapy). Both mainstream and unconventional medical practices are diverse and based on numerous different overlapping (and sometimes conflicting) under-standings of health and treatment. It is of interest that, in discussing the 'chiropractic paradigm', Coulter (1990) left it open as to whether chiropractic is its own unique paradigm, or consists of two or more paradigms or whether it is in fact a 'sub-paradigm' of naturopathy. Once more, the concept of a paradigm seems too flexible to be of explanatory value.

By requiring that complementary and conventional medicine are in themselves homogeneous, those who argue for the notion of separate paradigms tend to caricature what they claim to describe. Beinfield and Korngold (1995), for example, quoted Descartes to explain western medical thinking. St George (1994a) stated that, in conventional medicine, 'subjective influences on the body are excluded as irrelevant, reducing the body to an impersonal biomolecular machine'. In addition, treatment is based on the 'external engineering of (physicochemical) derangements by a doctor-scientist'. It is not at all clear how, say, general practice, hospice care, clinical psychology or nursing are based on Descartes, or reduce the body to a machine, utilize Beinfield and Korngold's conception of health care as a 'war on disease' or involve the external engineering of 'physicochemical derangements'. Crucially, no evidence is ever presented to justify these models of conventional and complementary medicine. This allows authors to become increasingly divorced from reality: Launsø (1994), for example, stated that, in conventional medicine, 'the placebo is defined as an evil to be fought against. How placebo effects are activated ... and with what consequence for the healing process have been of very little interest. In medical circles, the placebo has been considered uncontrollable, something the researcher had no power over: a Monster'. Placebo is no doubt an underexplored concept in medicine, but it is simply false to claim that conventional scientists consider it an evil to be fought against (e.g. see White, Tursky and Schwartz, 1985).

One of the most interesting features of these caricatures, and certainly the most important from the perspective of research, is the assertion that conventional medicine is only interested in objective changes and processes. Watson (1995), for example, stated that 'paradigm I science is structured to remove any human factors from the context of the study, setting up a model that is detached from feelings, meaning and subjective experiences'. Similarly, Mills (1986) asserted that 'current medical research generally concerns itself only with measuring events and data divorced from the human being', while St George (1994a) claimed, 'the subjectivity of doctor and the patient, as well as doctor/patient interactions, are understood to be irrelevant to therapy'. It is hard to see what evidence there is for such statements. Patient-assessed pain and anxiety are typical outcome measures in clinical trials. Both have at least something to do with feelings and subjective experiences. Similarly, it has been possible not only to conduct but to publish conventional clinical trials on techniques such as psychotherapy (e.g. Winston et al. 1994) and meditation (e.g. Dillbeck, 1977) in which the subjectivity of the patient is crucial to therapy. Moreover, it would surely be difficult to find any health care professional who believes that the interaction between doctor and patient is irrelevant. Again we see that reference to paradigms leads to crude generalizations rather than useful, detailed analysis.

Research methods are paradigm-specific

If the same research methods can be used across different paradigms, there would be no point in raising the issue of paradigms in the methodology debate. So even if it were to be argued that 'paradigm' was a coherent, meaningful and accurate generalization to apply to health care, a case would still need to made that, because a complementary therapy constitutes a different paradigm, it requires different research methods. This is perhaps the key issue in the methodological debate: to what extent are research methods paradigm-specific, i.e. applicable to only one paradigm?

Although no author has explicitly answered this question, many papers are heavy with the implication that different paradigms require different methodologies. Scheid (1993), for example, described conventional research methods as 'intellectually untenable' when applied to complementary medicine and called for 'forms of scholarship more appropriate to the tradition in which we work'. Launsø (1994) suggested that paradigms are seamless wholes such that methodologies may be deduced from therapies and therapies deduced from methodologies: 'the controlled clinical trial ... (is) an essential tool for the mechanistic-objectifying paradigm. The research object of this paradigm is the physical and measurable body ... a treatment can only be documented scientifically if it can be reduced to a technique'. The clinical trial (a research method) is seen to have resulted from a set of treatments (conventional medicine); the set of treatments is defined by the parameters of the research methods.

The belief that research methods are paradigm-specific is also implicit in statements which seem to call for complementary medicine to abandon conventional research techniques. As St George (1994a) put it: 'the time has come for complementary medicine to turn away from the need to obtain legitimacy from orthodox medicine by adopting its paradigm and research methods' and take the 'road to a new paradigm ... this *must* be the road that complementary medicine takes' (1994b). Or as Launsø (1994) summed up an analysis of research methodology: 'are we going to follow in the footsteps of established medical science ... or (do) we dare to blaze our own trail?'.

If research methods are paradigm-specific, it becomes difficult to explain the existence of randomized controlled trials on psychotherapy for personality disorder (e.g. Winston *et al.*, 1994) or on prayer (e.g. Byrd, 1988). In the former case, the therapy is not reduced to a technique and the research object is not the physical body; in the latter case, prayer can hardly be said to be typical of conventional treatments. Both of these trials provided useful information which supported the use of the technique in question. Controlled clinical trials (the 'tool for the mechanistic-objectifying paradigm') have been conducted on all sorts of therapies, practised in all sorts of ways.

Moreover, if complementary medicine is a different paradigm, and if a different paradigm requires different research methods, we need to know the constituents of the new methods. Interestingly, proponents of new paradigm research rarely do spell out any genuinely new methodologies. Launsø (1994) argued that research is needed to 'develop and explicate scientific paradigms for conducting research on alternative therapy', but no further details are given. Watson (1995) cited numerous methodological papers to support contentions such as that 'nursing scholarship outside the modern science paradigm is now generally accepted', but does not refer to a single example of primary research, i.e. research in which something was discovered by using new methods. However, when authors do state the methodologies that they would like to see used, these do not generally constitute a 'new paradigm'. St George (1994a), for example, called for a focus on basic science and applied health services research including clinical audit and cost-effectiveness studies. Similarly, Korr (1991) stated the case for medical outcome studies on osteopathy and Coulter (1993) argued for qualitative research to complement quantitative methods. Reason (1988) is rare in that he has described a genuinely novel set of research methods and has presented original data resulting from their use. That said, it is unlikely that Reason's 'cooperative inquiry' will be able to answer more than a subset of questions pertinent in complementary medicine research (see below). If research methods are indeed paradigm-specific, and if conventional research designs are therefore inappropriate to complementary medicine, it seems that there is little to replace them.

Those working within a paradigm are unable to look outside it

A number of authors support the view that paradigms are like separate, sealed, mirrored rooms from which light neither escapes nor enters. 'Biomedical research' stated St George (1994a) 'is conservative research which supports current orthodoxy'. Launsø (1994) went further: 'if the healing process were in fact subject-dependent, the fact would not be recognized as it would threaten the goal of the scientific activity'. This seems to suggest that scientists are so blinded by their assumptions that they are unable to see outside of them.

It is relatively obvious that prior assumptions and theories can act as a constraint and this seems to be an inevitable and necessary part of research. For example, epidemiologists trying to determine why the rate of lung cancer increased following the Second World War formed hypotheses in the light of their understanding of pathology. They reasoned that lung cancer might result from inhalation of a carcinogenic substance and therefore investigated smoking and tarmac rather than sexual behaviour, alcohol use, racial origin or astrological birth sign. These assumptions speeded up the process of coming to useful conclusions about the cause of lung cancer. Sometimes assumptions have been unhelpful and sometimes they have been misleading. A classic example in complementary medicine research was the assumption that needling of incorrect acupuncture locations does not have a therapeutic effect (Gaw, Chang and Shaw, 1975).

However, it is surely false to claim that any group, even 'mechanistic-objectifying' scientists, is inherently unable to recognize and reflect critically on its assumptions. One of the more unusual aspects of some of the writing about paradigms is that, in order to give examples of that which is outside orthodoxy, reference is often made to conventional theories and mainstream research. Data on psychoneuro-immunology or the placebo effect might be cited to support the importance of the mind-body link, or studies linking electromagnetic emissions to leukaemia referenced to support energy medicine.

Even where authors do not make explicit reference to mainstream science, it is rare that a proposed limitation of the biomedical paradigm is not a recognized part of medical practice. For example, St George (1994a) claimed that medical science views disease as 'caused by specific physicochemical derangements'. This is not always the case. There is even a name ('functional disorders') for diseases which do not have a physical basis. Similarly, Beinfield and Korngold's (1995) assertion that the biomechanical model requires that reality be 'reduced into smaller and smaller discrete constituents', seems to ignore that the limits to reductionism is a lively debate in human and animal behaviour (Rose, Lewontin and Kamin, 1984). Medical science does involve assumptions, but it seems untrue to state that it is impossible to look outside of them.

Paradigms are universal and there can only be one at a time: the current medical paradigm is outdated and is about to be replaced

Reason (1988) claimed that 'the old world-view, with its fragmented and alienated mechanical metaphors, is discarded as we move in to a participatory universe'. Watson (1995) described an 'evolution of scientific inquiry' starting with Paradigm I (particulate-deterministic) said to be dominant until the 1960s; Paradigm II (interactive-integrative) said to be dominant during the last two to three decades and the forthcoming Paradigm III (unitary-transformative). Coulter (1993) cited those who believe that the 'biomedical paradigm' should be replaced by a 'holistic paradigm'. St George (1994a) used more explicitly Kuhnian language in stating that he personally believes that a 'paradigm-shift is really taking place'. In sum, we are in the midst of, about to undergo, or in need of a change of paradigms. Stable as they seem, the current understandings of health, and how to research it, are about to be replaced.

The prospect of paradigm shift within medicine is deeply problematic. Kuhn originally introduced the concept of paradigm to explain scientific, not medical, change. There is an important difference between health care and science. In science, it is generally only possible to have one paradigm at a time: there cannot be both Aristotelian and Gallilean cosmology, both phlogiston and oxygen or both evolution and creationism. In health care, the concurrent presence of two or more paradigms is not only possible, but desirable, and the stated aim of numerous providers: the surgeon works alongside the hospital chaplain and the general practitioner alongside the social worker. Interdisciplinary care, where health professionals from a number of different disciplines work together, is sometimes seen as the ideal form of patient care.

There is, however, a more profound problem with the notion of paradigm change: what evidence is there that it is taking place? Authors such as St George, Reason or Watson tend merely to assert that we are moving towards a new paradigm. They may quote other commentators or, rarely, provide examples of phenomena or research methods said to characterize the coming scientific order. But no data of significant sociological change are ever provided. If Reason is right that the old world-view is being discarded, or if Watson is correct in consigning the particulate-deterministic paradigm to the 1960s, they should be able to provide evidence (or at least suggest some possible sources). They could, for instance, analyse the activities of grant-making bodies to show a radical shift away from funding randomized clinical trials and towards funding new paradigm research. Alternatively, they could provide figures showing a shift of newly qualified doctors from surgery to therapeutic touch. No such examples are forthcoming. I would argue that this is because a paradigm shift is clearly not taking place. The last 20–30 years have seen the development of a number of interesting and valuable new ideas about medicine and methodology. These have added to rather than replaced existing understandings of health care.

The methodologies of the orthodox paradigm have had adverse effects on health and society: these methodologies are nothing less than tools of oppression

Writers on paradigms often make liberal use of powerful language to describe conventional methodology. St George (1994a) equates scientific advancement with 'an aggressive, invasive form of probing, dissection and analysis into a soul-less world of space, time, matter and forces (in which) a human being (becomes) an accidental arrangement of molecules in an impersonal "dead" universe'. Launsø (1994) asserted that the 'controlled clinical trial (is a) tool for regulating the development of an illness consciousness and actions that are fragmented', something which 'requires a passive body' and the use of treatments which 'maintain . . . passivity'. Reason (1988) stated that conventional research techniques are fragmenting, hierarchical, patriarchal and dominating and lead not only to the alienation of subjects but may be the root cause of ecological devastation, spiritual impoverishment and the breakdown of society. In contrast, the paradigm of research recommended by Reason is: 'holistic and unitary', it encourages 'empathy, responsibility and authentic colla-boration' and engenders the establishment of relationships and 'mutual love and concern'. Mills (1986) explicitly links conventional research to oppression in stating that, 'those of us concerned with protecting our therapies from unnecessary encroachment and control . . . (require) new models of research'. St George (1994b) went further: biomedical research requires a 'complete submission to the orthodox medical paradigm' possibly leading to 'the take-over of complementary medicine by orthodox doctors' and 'a distortion of its [complementary medicine's] essential nature in order to . . . fit into the needs and vested interests of orthodox medicine'. Scheid (1993) claimed that 'the scientific re-evaluation of traditional systems of medicine . . . amounts to acts of epistemological violence'.

These attacks provide further evidence that the notion of a paradigm is a tool against discourse. If you seriously wish to create a dialogue with someone, you do not normally start by claiming that they are aggressive, violent, self-interested and use techniques which have led to the breakdown of society. But such attacks also provide an insight into the thought processes behind much of the writing on paradigms. The paradigm argument in complementary medicine research seems to be engendered by a fear of the Other: dark forces representing beliefs to which the author does not subscribe will act to bring about ends which the author does not want to see. The paradigm moves from being an explanation for the nature of scientific change, to becoming the 'bogeyman': a packaging of nebulous fears and animosities into a discrete entity which no-one can see but whose existence can be deduced by its effects.

Paradigms lost: towards pluralism

In 1988, Reason published a collection of studies which utilized what he had previously described as 'new paradigm' research methods. The book begins with a quotation: 'If you have not lived through something, it is not true'. The question is, does it not depend on the something? Take lung cancer: to understand the human experience of lung cancer, its meaning, symbolism, fears and pains, one must live through it. But to understand what causes lung cancer, or how it may be diagnosed, personal contact and experience is not strictly necessary. So it may be more accurate to say: 'If you have not lived through some things, then they are not true in some ways'.

Reason went on to describe a 'cooperative inquiry' which sets out to explore the concept of holistic medicine. The information that this inquiry produces is extremely valuable, particularly given that the concept of 'holism' has tended to be used without any real understanding of its meaning. But the elucidation of professional practice and theory is surely not the only purpose of inquiry. For example, Reason's research suggested that using a wide range of interventions is one aspect of holistic medical practice. What if we want to know exactly which interventions to use and which to avoid? It is unlikely that we could depend solely on Reason's cooperative inquiry.

In 1993, a group of midwives started prescribing lavender oil to women after childbirth, a practice which is recommended by aromatherapists for healing the perineum (e.g. Lawless, 1994). A survey revealed that 85% of women thought that the remedy had been of benefit. Presumably, if we had conducted a cooperative inquiry with patients and practitioners we would have come to the conclusion that lavender oil is considered to be a valuable intervention. However, a recent randomized controlled trial, conducted by the midwives involved and using the lavender precisely as suggested by aromatherapists, found no difference between real lavender oil and a synthetic lavender preparation (Dale and Cornwell, 1994). In this instance, blinding and randomization eliminated what turned out to be a human bias in trying to evaluate the benefits of lavender oil.

Cooperative enquiry is a useful addition to the range of techniques available to researchers. It is not a replacement for them. It may be that we will never improve practice, or understand novel concepts such as holistic medicine or power sharing between patient and practitioner, without techniques such as Reason's cooperative inquiry-style research. But it is equally unlikely that we will ever generate reliable information about the efficacy of therapies without at least some randomized controlled trials, or understand dangers in our environment (such as smoking) without traditional epidemiological techniques.

This leads us to my central point. It is nonsensical to talk about the appropriateness of research methods without reference to the *question* being asked in research (e.g. see Vickers, 1996). Few of the authors discussing paradigms sufficiently emphasize the importance of focusing on a particular question and then matching a research design to the question. Research methods seem to be tied to paradigms, rather than questions. Certain questions do only make sense within a particular medical system (e.g. what forms of needle manipulation are most appropriate for dissipating excess Qi?), but it is still the question, rather than the paradigm, which drives the research design. It is this issue of questions which reveals both the strengths and weaknesses of 'new paradigm' thinking.

On the plus side, those authors who use the concept of the paradigm have done well to articulate some of the limitations of orthodox research methodology. It is hard, for example, to disagree with Reason (1988) when he points out that the conventional distinction between the subject and object of research causes problems in some contexts. A good example might be understanding the problems of disadvantaged groups, where it is seems only right that members of those groups should partake in setting the research agenda. Similarly, St George (1994a) is surely right to call for applied health services research in complementary medicine. One might also be sympathetic to some of the critiques of conventional medicine which have been offered. Many would agree that conventional medicine has often overemphasized objective statements about individual body parts at the expense of how patients feel as a whole. Furthermore, it is worth reminding ourselves that we do not live in a simple, single, objective reality; rather, there are various ways of looking at the world and it is sometimes difficult to translate ideas across these different perspectives.

The great weakness of 'paradigms' in the methodological debate on complementary medicine is that they have been of so little practical value. Writers have predicated arguments on an obscure and imprecise concept, used esoteric and impenetrable language and employed strong rhetoric to caricature and denounce conventional medicine and research techniques. Practical advice to a researcher interested in complementary medicine is hard to find. It is interesting that Peter Reason, the one author who has both developed practical ideas on research methodology and who has undertaken genuinely useful research (e.g. Reason 1991, 1995; Reason et al., 1992) has abandoned the term 'new paradigm research' and now speaks of cooperative inquiry. In fact, the term 'paradigm' rarely appears in Reason's later work at all. There appears to be an inverse correlation between discussion of paradigms and the production of useful research results and practical ideas on methodology.

In conclusion, would it really be a good thing if health care switched to a subject-oriented paradigm or if the 'old world-view' were to be discarded? We would first have to find out whether the subject-oriented paradigm will solve all our problems (even in acute medicine) and whether there is anything useful in conventional methodology. But it is unnecessary to do so. We do not need a 'paradigm-shift', rather we could aim to incorporate new ideas, where appropriate, and to expand existing theory and practice, where it is useful to do so. It is surely time to foster discourse and incorporate different points of view and to abandon the forced choice between different, global systems. In short, we need to stop talking about paradigms and to start embracing pluralism.

References

Beinfield, H. and Korngold, E. (1995) Chinese traditional medicine: an introductory overview. *Alternative Therapies in Health and Medicine*, **1**, 44–52

Byrd, R. (1988) Positive therapeutic effects of intercessory prayer in a coronary care unit population. *Southern Medical Journal*, **91**, 826–829

Coulter, I. D. (1990) The chiropractic paradigm. *Journal of Manipulative and Physiological Therapeutics*, **13**, 279–287

Coulter, I. D. (1993) Alternative philosophical and investigatory paradigms for chiropractic. *Journal of Manipulative and Physiological Therapeutics*, **16**, 419–425

Dale, A. and Cornwell, S. (1994) The role of lavender oil in relieving perineal discomfort following childbirth: a blind, randomised clinical trial. *Journal of Advanced Nursing*, **19**, 89–96

Dillbeck, M. C. (1977) The effect of the Transcendental Meditation technique on anxiety level. *Journal of Clinical Psychology*, **33**, 1076–1078

Gaw, A. C., Chang, L. W. and Shaw, L.-C. (1975) Efficacy of acupuncture on osteoarthritic pain. A controlled, double-blind study. *New England Journal of Medicine*, **293**, 37–38

Korr, I. M. (1991) Osteopathic research: the needed paradigm shift. *Journal of the American Osteopathy Association*, **91**, 156–171

Kuhn, T. S. (1962) *The Structure of Scientific Revolutions*. Chicago: Chicago University Press

Lakatos, I. and Musgrave, A. (eds.) (1965) *Criticism and the Growth of Knowledge*. Cambridge: Cambridge University Press

Launsø, L. (1994) How to kiss a monster. In: *Studies in Alternative Therapy 1*, edited by H. Johannessen, L. Launsø, S. Gosvigolesen and F. Stangård. Denmark: Odense University Press

Lawless, J. (1994) *Lavender Oil*. London: Thorsons

Masarsky, C. S. and Weber, M. (1991) Stop paradigm erosion. *Journal of Manipulative and Physiological Therapeutics*, **14**, 323–326

Masterman, M. (1965) The nature of a paradigm. In: *Criticism and the Growth of Knowledge*, edited by I. Lakatos and A. Musgrave. Cambridge: Cambridge University Press

Mills, S. (1986) Conflicting research needs in complementary medicine. *Complementary Medicine Research*, **1**, 40–47

Nagel, E. (1961) *The Structure of Science*. New York: Harcourt, Brace and Ward

National Institutes for Health (1994) *Alternative Medicine: Expanding Medical Horizons*. NIH Publication no 94–066

Reason, P. (ed.) (1988) *Human Inquiry in Action*. London: Sage

Reason, P. (1991) Power and conflict in multidisciplinary collaboration. *Complementary Medicine Research*, **5**, 144–150

Reason, P. (1995) Complementary practice at Phoenix Surgery: first steps in cooperative inquiry. *Complementary Therapy and Medicine*, **3**, 37–41

Reason, P., Chase, H. D., Desser, A., Melhuish, C., Morrison, S., Peters, D. *et al.*

(1992) Towards a clinical framework for collaboration between general and complementary practitioners: discussion paper. *Journal of the Royal Society of Medicine*, **85**, 161–169

Rose, S., Lewontin, R. C., and Kamin, L. J. (1984). *Not in Our Genes*. London: Penguin

Rubik, B. (1994) The perennial challenge of anomalies at the frontiers of science. *British Homoeopathic Journal*, **83**, 155–166

Scheid, V. (1993) Orientalism revisited. *European Journal of Oriental Medicine*, **1**, 23–33

St George, D. (1994a) Towards a research and development strategy for complementary medicine. *The Homoeopath*, **54**, 254–256

St George, D. (1994b) Research and development in herbal medicine: biomedical research or new paradigm? *European Journal of Herbal Medicine*, **1**, 38–39

Vickers, A. J. (1996) Methodological issues in complementary and alternative medicine research: a personal reflection on 10 years of debate in the UK. *Journal of Alternative and Complementary Medicine*, (in press)

Watson, J. (1995) Nursing's caring-healing paradigm as exemplar for alternative medicine? *Alternative Therapies in Health and Medicine*, **1**, 64–69

White, L., Tursky, B. and Schwartz, G. E. (1985) *Placebo: Theory, Research and Mechanisms*. New York: The Guildford Press

Winston, A., Laikin, M., Pollack, J., Samstag, L. W., McCullough, L. and Muran, J. C. (1994) Short-term psychotherapy of personality disorders. *American Journal of Psychiatry*, **151**, 190–194

Chapter 2

Research methodologies in complementary medicine: making sure it works

Karl-Ludwig Resch and Edzard Ernst

Introduction

Research in complementary medicine (alternative medicine) shares a vital objective with research in mainstream medicine (conventional medicine, orthodox medicine), i.e. trying to find reliable and valid answers to the question of the likelihood or the extent of benefit our next patient with a given condition can expect from a certain diagnostic technique or intervention. Since this objective demands the establishment of a causal relationship between the diagnostic technique or intervention (exposure) and the outcome (effect) (Elwood, 1988), research methodologies in complementary medicine must follow, in principle, the same formal rules as research methodologies in mainstream medicine, where there are well-established research methodologies, particularly focusing on quantitative research (Schlesselman, 1982; Elwood, 1988; Gelijns, 1990; Sackett *et al.*, 1991; Mays and Pope, 1995). This chapter reviews general formal requirements for medical research before focusing on specific problems of research in complementary medicine.

From ideas to evidence

Qualitative research

Any research activity needs some form of initiation. It is often triggered by curiosity about a personal or a reported observation (case report), which is deemed unexpected but not irrelevant (Figure 2.1). Once attention is drawn to a certain phenomenon, a thorough search of the literature (including the 'grey' literature) followed by careful consideration of the existing evidence (Vickers, 1995) is the obligatory initial activity and the most promising strategy against bias and confounding at this early stage. Depending on the existing evidence, hypothesis-generating research is the usual next step. It is

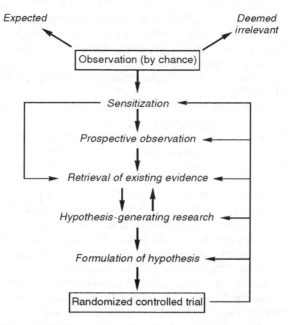

Figure 2.1 Sequence of activities from a clinical observation to causal evidence

referred to as qualitative research and includes single case studies, retrospective studies, surveys of all kinds, open, uncontrolled, and/or non-randomized prospective trials (Elwood, 1988).

Qualitative research methods are appropriate to assess, for instance, prevalence, attitudes, demand, time trends or belief systems in order to enhance our knowledge of an area of interest, and to provide a proper basis to formulate a hypothesis. This type of research, however, does not provide any firm evidence on causal relationships. Qualitative research methods have their own methodology which will not be detailed here (for further reading a recent series in the *British Medical Journal* can be recommended) (Mays and Pope, 1995).

It should be mentioned that 'pilot trials' also fall into this category. They are often helpful or even indispensable in addressing qualitatively areas that have previously been unresearched.

Quantitative research

Quantitative research aims at hypothesis testing and, typically, at evaluating the efficacy, safety, and (cost-)effectiveness of diagnosis and therapy. An investigation into efficacy would normally be the first step, where efficacy is referred to as the probability or extent of benefits under ideal conditions of use or the potential benefit inherent in an exposure (Gelijns and Thier, 1990). Once there is evidence for a positive answer concerning efficacy, the question would arise whether the exposure is safe or what its potential for harm is, i.e. the relation of risk and benefit.

Positive evidence on the issues of efficacy and safety would then open the way to a more pragmatic approach, i.e. an investigation into the effectiveness of the exposure, where effectiveness refers to the benefits under average conditions of use (Gelijns and Thier, 1990). A highly efficacious exposure does not necessarily have to be highly effective as well. Imagine a tea with a powerful potential to alleviate a certain ailment, which tasted so bitter that hardly anybody would be prepared to use it. Finally, an intervention or a diagnostic method would not only have to be effective and safe in order to become a relevant new feature in health care, it would also have to be affordable. Depending on the point of view, this question would be addressed by cost-effectiveness, cost-benefit, or cost-utility studies.

All these aspects are independent of knowledge or awareness of the nature, i.e. the mechanisms or the mode of action, of an exposure which, although interesting and to some extent helpful to optimize efficacy, safety and/or effectiveness of an exposure, are not an essential feature of clinical research.

Quantitative research without a proper basis (e.g. through qualitative research) is not only a waste of time, money and labour, it is also deeply unethical, because it unnecessarily involves volunteers or patients in clinical trials (with no prospect of success) (Altman, 1994).

Methodological requirements

Not only have the evidence levels of the different research strategies and their sequence to be borne in mind, but some methodological requirements are almost an essential precondition in order to be able to generate reliable and valid findings (Andersen, 1990).

Study period and sample size

Study period and sample size must be adequate to allow a potential effect to become evident. For ethical as well as for statistical and economic reasons, the sample size should neither be larger nor smaller than necessary; proper sample size calculations are therefore mandatory (Altman, 1980).

Bias and confounding

The definition of meaningful inclusion and exclusion criteria aims at making the sample more homogeneous and, by reducing the 'background noise', at increasing the power of the study. Once again, every effort must be made to minimize the risk that bias or confounding factors spoil the results (Elwood, 1988).

There are two major sources of bias: selection bias, which addresses the problem of inadequate recruitment procedures; and information bias which results from inadequate or invalid data assessment, thereby negatively affecting the (internal) validity of a study. A confounder is defined as a third extraneous factor which satisfies both the condition and the effect counterfeiting a causal link between them, where in fact the relation is only spurious. An often cited example is the spurious relation between the prevalence of 'yellow' fingertips and lung cancer. The underlying causal factor would be cigarette smoking, and it is obvious that careful manicure could not be an appropriate intervention to prevent lung cancer.

Main outcome parameter

In clinical research the main outcome parameter should, whenever possible, be a clinical rather than a surrogate endpoint. It should have a reasonably good sensitivity and specificity, and the method should be valid (which includes good reproducibility and acceptable precision). Commonly available and frequently used methods are to be given preference over 'exotic' or 'self-made' ones. This also makes pooling of results in systematic reviews (or meta-analyses) more effective. Continuous variables incorporate considerably more information than ordinal or nominal ones, an aspect that greatly affects sample size or study power. The intention-to-treat principle is crucial for studies aiming at effectiveness (intervention effects under 'everyday life' conditions), but less important if efficacy (intervention effects under optimal conditions) is under investigation. Nevertheless, the likelihood of factors other than chance as a motive to drop out has to be considered thoroughly.

Establishing causality

Randomized controlled trials

Besides a sound methodology as outlined in the previous paragraph, hypothesis testing ('establishing causality') requires two fundamental preconditions: proper randomization and a control condition ('randomized controlled trial', 'RCT'). While the former is a formal requirement technically relatively easy to be realized (Schlesselman, 1982), the latter profits considerably from the know-how and medical experience of the investigator.

The necessity of controls is obvious since any comment on an exposure being 'as effective as' or 'more effective than' demands a second sample for comparison. The rationale for randomization is somewhat more complex.

Randomization

When a patient presents with a certain condition (i.e. a disease, a symptom, an ailment, a complaint) and is given a certain treatment, any changes observed are likely to be linked to the intervention under clinical conditions. This, however, is a simplistic view that does not take into consideration other factors which could very well have contributed to or be the real cause of the observed changes (Figure 2.2).

Relatively well known and appreciated, although insufficiently studied to date, are the so-called non-specific effects or placebo

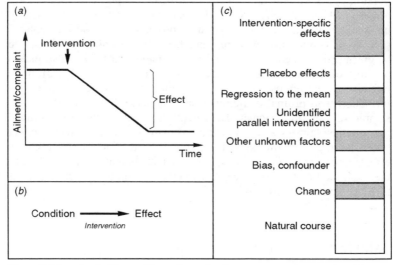

Figure 2.2 Perceived effects: effects observed subsequent to an intervention (*a*) are likely to be seen as a consequence of the intervention (*b*). However, many factors other than the intervention (*c*) could have contributed to or be the true causal factors, since they all sum up to the 'perceived effect'

effects, which include the phenomena of transference/counter-transference and expectation (Ernst and Resch, 1995a). It has been shown that these effects can account for a major part of the clinically apparent effect.

A statistician would point out the relevance of the phenomenon of regression to the mean (Schlesselman, 1982), which includes the assumption that patients are likely to present with their complaint at a 'relative maximum' which could consequently be expected to regress in due course due to its natural fluctuation around an individual mean.

Certainly the natural course of the condition must not be underestimated, since most conditions have a tendency to get better even without any intervention. Patients might apply other measures, which might have been suggested by friends, the lay press, or exploratory reading, or could be based on previous experience, to treat their condition – measures of which the observer might not be aware. Finally, chance, bias and confounder and, most likely, other still unknown factors may relevantly have influenced the observed changes (Elwood, 1988; Andersen, 1990).

Thus, it becomes obvious that causality of one factor to the observed effect can only be established to the extent that one succeeds in keeping it free from contamination with any other factor. This requires holding all factors constant across groups except for the factor under investigation which can only be achieved if patients are allocated strictly at random into the different arms (Figure 2.3).

It should be mentioned that all these different potential factors are far from being independent from each other, but might rather have complex interactions: increasing the impact of one factor might be at the expense of one or various others. These problems are poorly understood and certainly under-researched to date. Nevertheless they can be controlled for by proper randomization (see Chapter 3).

Controls

It is, however, not just the qualitative aspect of the sheer presence of a control group; the choice of an *appropriate* control condition has to be considered very carefully too (Ross and Charlotte, 1951). It is crucially dependent on the main objective of the study, e.g. testing of the overall efficacy/effectiveness of an intervention, of specific versus non-specific effects, or of the relative efficacy/effectiveness of alternative or additional interventions. This in turn determines the level of rigour of the blinding strategy needed (single, double, triple blind).

'Placebo' as the control intervention is ethically acceptable only if there is no 'gold standard' intervention available which causally

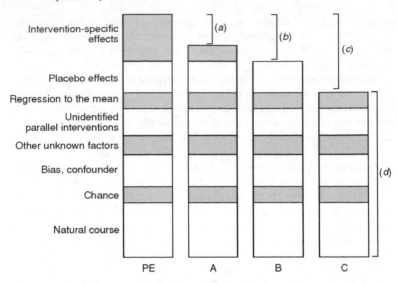

Figure 2.3 Rationale of the randomized controlled trial: changes of an outcome variable over time ('perceived effects', PE) might have been caused by one or a combination of various factors, not necessarily including any intervention-specific effects. To establish a causal role of the latter the changes of the outcome variable over time in a control group have to be compared to those in the intervention group (PE). Typically, the control group could be a group receiving another specific intervention (*a*), a placebo intervention (*b*), or no treatment (*c*). Randomization and study design would have to assure that (*d*) can be assumed not to differ between groups, otherwise (*a*), (*b*), or (*c*) could not be considered a valid finding

interferes with the underlying condition. In this case it would be irrelevant simply to demonstrate that an alternative approach 'works'; it would have to be superior to the established standard in terms of efficacy, safety or cost.

Ethical considerations also determine the potential inclusion of an 'untreated' control group, although its presence is crucial if non-specific effects are to be quantified besides specific effects (Ernst and Resch, 1995a). Feasibility is another important *de facto* criterion. The more a study aims at breaking new ground the less specific an approach should be chosen in order to avoid false-negative results.

Strategies to define a control group

Cross-sectional comparisons of two groups in a longitudinal study require roughly twice as many participants as cross-over studies which, in turn, exclusively suit investigations of 'symptomatic' interventions which clearly do not causally affect or even cure the underlying disease or condition. In addition, cross-over studies are burdened with other problems such as carry-over effects. A 'matched-pairs' analysis aims at combining the advantages of both approaches at the expense of being, strictly speaking, not a randomized study (Schlesselman, 1982).

Limitations of 'N-of-1' trials

Although a helpful tool to study the respective efficacy of different treatment regimens for a particular patient (Guyatt et al., 1988), 'N-of-1' trials cannot provide information beyond the given single case. Whether pooling of a reasonably large number of N-of-1 trials is statistically appropriate remains to be shown (Campbell, 1994). Formal considerations do not suggest that pooling can lead to information comparable to the one derived from a randomized controlled trial, because the intention of the N-of-1 trial is information on a particular patient and therefore the criterion of random selection is not fulfilled. Technically, a 'meta-analysis of N-of-1 trials' is a 'retrospective case series' of independent individualized (multiple) cross-over trials.

Specific features of complementary medicine research

Holistic versus reductionistic

An attribute commonly used in connection with complementary medicine is 'holistic', whereas orthodox medicine (research) is often termed 'reductionistic'. This might be true for particular areas of biomedical research, especially 'basic research', but the clinician is typically interested in the impact of his intervention strategy on the patient. In turn, basic science in complementary medicine might find a reductionistic approach as useful as orthodox medicine to gain insights gradually into a matter that might be far too complex to be tackled otherwise. Therefore, it does not seem justified to use the terms holistic/reductionistic to differentiate between mainstream medicine and complementary medicine; it should rather be used to describe different investigational approaches within each of the two fields of medicines. The impression that the proportion of holistic versus reductionistic approaches is different between orthodox and complementary medicine does not confirm the notion of a concep-tional difference between the two, but reflects the fact that they primarily focus on different areas of the 'basic human condition of illness and disease' (McGouty, 1993), as, for instance, life-threatening emergencies and pain management/quality of life in chronic incurable diseases respectively.

It has repeatedly been stressed that the 'reductionist approach' of a clinical trial is unsuitable to test the 'subtle' effects of 'holistic' medicine (Patel, 1987). This claim does not seem to be true nor ethically acceptable; every individual patient has the right to receive the most beneficial treatment or the treatment that prospectively offers the best chance to be effective. Therefore, if effects are 'too subtle' to be recognizable (e.g. through using quality of life, well-being, or patient preference as an outcome measure), can they honestly be considered relevant? Similar considerations would apply to the argument of 'long-term effects', if those effects take unacceptably long to become evident. However, if a complementary medicine approach reasonably claims to cure or alleviate a condition only over a long period of time, and no comparable or more effective alternative is at hand, it might be worthwhile considering undertaking a randomized controlled trial long enough to gain new insights. In any case, it must be ensured that any potential disadvantages for patients, for instance, due to not receiving another potentially useful therapy during their participation in the trial, are kept at an ethically acceptable minimum.

Main outcome parameter

With research in complementary medicine certain methodological problems appear to be more prevalent and relevant than in mainstream medicine, especially the lack of a simple, established, readily 'measurable' physical or biochemical correlate (surrogate) (Patel, 1987; Mercer, Long and Smith, 1995). Sometimes the seriousness of a disease might not be readily recognizable by a patient (e.g. early stages of malignant or infectious diseases) and therefore a medically trained specialist might focus on an outcome parameter, the relevance of which is not fully transparent to the patient. If, however, the intervention aims at alleviating symptoms rather than claiming to interfere causally with the underlying disease, a 'symptomatic variable' seems justified as the main outcome measurement (e.g. pain, quality of life, well-being).

In practice, many complementary therapies consist of a complex composition of different components; this, however, is not specific to complementary medicine. Here research mainly requires 'clinical common sense' in choosing an adequate design and a meaningful main outcome parameter. Moreover, it is argued that complementary therapies are 'holistic' and thus cannot be pressed into the framework of reductionistic research; this notion is only valid if an inappropriate outcome parameter is chosen. Given the right outcome measure even the most holistic approach can be evaluated through randomized controlled trials.

Control intervention

Often there is no genuine 'placebo intervention' available, i.e. potential control interventions differ in more than just the lack of the 'specific component'. The hypothesis must take into account what can be controlled for and what cannot. Often an 'indistinguishable' control intervention is not feasible (e.g. in aromatherapy or manipulation), but its differences from the intervention can certainly be minimized. One could, for instance, try to use a dummy intervention with a similar non-specific impact (the validity of this assumption might have to be assessed by means of pilot trials); an intervention could be applied 'optimally' versus 'poorly'; an additional impressive dummy variable could be given to both groups in order to distract the attention away from the intervention under investigation.

Some complementary therapies are based on concepts that differ considerably from 'biomedical concepts' (e.g. homoeopathy, Ayurveda, traditional Chinese medicine), thus requiring an adaptation of the 'classic' randomized controlled trial. If not yet available, proper adaptations are not impossible *per se* but would have to be developed and tested (Högel, Walach and Gaus, 1994; Ernst and Resch, 1995b).

Discussion

Denying the necessity to scrutinize complementary medicine would mean to accept readily any claim, however far fetched or even dangerous, as soon as it is labelled complementary medicine. Within complementary medicine, different contradictory, theoretical and conceptual frameworks exist. Thus it becomes obvious that not all of them can be true, at least not at one time and for a given problem. Besides the immensely complex problem of research into the theoretical concepts and conceptional frameworks, proper research into efficacy and effectiveness aims at providing a potential future patient with a greater likelihood of receiving better treatment from somebody somewhere. If it were clear that the therapeutic intervention is not related to the observed effect, it would not make sense to apply it in order to achieve this effect.

It can be assumed that patients who seek help from one form of complementary medicine have frequently been treated unsuccessfully by mainstream medicine and other forms of complementary medicine. They might therefore represent a rather selected subsample of a population of patients with a certain condition, from which one cannot possibly generalize that a certain complementary medicine intervention is ineffective in principle, if yet another therapeutic attempt was unsuccessful. Thus the lack of proof of efficacy is not necessarily the proof of lack of efficacy. 'Perceived failure' could furthermore be due to the wrong question (looking in the wrong direction), the wrong instrument (the use of a microscope instead of a telescope), or an incompetently performed investigation (insufficient skills in handling the methodology).

The vast majority of forms of complementary medicine have at least one essential feature in common with mainstream medicine, i.e. their underlying principles as well as their practical performance is taught in 'schools'. This implies that the respective skills are thought to be suitable to produce, under certain circumstances, a predictable effect. Both complementary medicine and mainstream medicine therapists are confident that they have something in their respective therapeutic arsenals that can help a future patient better than something else or no treatment at all. These two very 'pragmatic assumptions' have 'scientific synonyms': reproducibility and causality. It becomes obvious that, although sometimes put in question, these two aspects are essential features of any medicine, whether mainstream or complementary. The real debate seems thus more a discussion on the 'right way' than on the ultimate target, in other words a discussion on which outcome measure is most appropriate or justified.

It has been stated that there is a 'significant gap between the "stronger" (and more quantitative) methods preferred by orthodox medicine and the "weaker" (and more qualitative) methods associated with complementary therapies' (Mercer, Long and Smith, 1995). This could be attributable to the concept of orthodox medicine and complementary therapies representing 'two different worlds'. Interestingly, it could also be applied to describe 'established' fields versus 'less established' fields in mainstream medicine as, for instance, immunology and physiotherapy. It holds true, too, if the present state of 'established' fields is compared to their historic state (e.g. decades or a century ago). In other words, there could be a close relation between academic representation and, in consequence, research sources and research skills on the one hand and the preferred scientific approach on the other.

To 'facilitate collaborative research between patient and therapist rather than research on patients' was claimed an issue 'to be considered when undertaking research into complementary therapies' (Mercer, Long and Smith, 1995). Again, this sort of research cannot provide any reliable information about the effectiveness and usefulness of a certain therapeutic intervention beyond a particular patient treated by a particular therapist. It is therefore of limited help for other patients to be treated by another therapist.

Another argument often raised is that concerns about the benefit of each individual patient do not allow putting patients at risk of receiving a 'dummy' treatment. One could respond that it is clearly much less ethical to withhold forever potential advances in treatment from all future patients, which would be the consequence of studying open questions inadequately (e.g. by not applying a dummy treatment to a limited number of patients).

Conclusion and prospects

In conclusion, research methodologies in complementary medicine should meet all conventional methodological requirements and, in addition, those of the modalities that are being tested. Any approach could be appropriate depending on the research question, but causal evidence can only come from randomized controlled trials (Elwood, 1988; Sheldon, 1994). However, adaptations of existing designs and/or development of new investigational strategies (Gaus and Högel, 1995) as well as new and 'unconventional' outcome measures are often needed (*Lancet*, 1995). This is a challenge to be met with methodological skills, experience, creativity, and even fantasy.

References

Altman, G. (1980) How large a sample? *British Medical Journal*, **281**, 1336–1338

Altman, D. G. (1994) The scandal of poor medical research. *British Medical Journal*, **308**, 283–284

Andersen, B. (1990) *Methodological Errors in Medical Research*. Oxford: Blackwell

Campbell, M. J. (1994) Commentary: N of 1 trials may be useful for informed decision making. *British Medical Journal*, **309**, 1045–1046

Elwood, J. M. (1988) *Causal Relationships in Medicine*. Oxford: Oxford University Press

Ernst, E. and Resch, K. L. (1995a) Concept of true and perceived placebo effects. *British Medical Journal*, **311**, 551–553

Ernst, E. and Resch, K. L. (1995b) The 'Optional cross-over design' for randomized controlled trials. *Fundamental and Clinical Pharmacology*, **9**, 508–511.

Gaus, W. and Högel, J. (1995) Studies on the efficacy of unconventional therapies. *Drug Research*, **45**, 88–92

Gelijns, A. C. (ed.). (1990) *Modern Methods of Clinical Investigation*. Washington, DC: National Academy Press

Gelijns, A. C. and Thier, S. O. (1990) Medical technology development: an introduction to the innovation-evaluation nexus. In: *Modern Methods of Clinical Investigation*, edited by A. C. Gelijns. Washington, DC: National Academy Press. pp. 1–15

Guyatt, G., Sackett, D., Taylor, D. W., Chong, J., Roberts, R. and Pugsley, S. (1986) Determining optimal therapy – randomized trials in individual patients. *New England Journal of Medicine*, **314**, 889–892

Högel, J., Walach, H. and Gaus, W. (1994) Change-to-open-label design. Proposal and discussion of a new design for parallel-group double-masked trials. *Drug Resource*, **44**, 97–99

Lancet. (1995) Editorial. Quality of life and clinical trials. **ii**, 1–2

McGouty, H. (1993) How to evaluate complementary therapies. A literature review. *Observatory Report Series no. 13*. Liverpool: Liverpool Public Health Authority

Mays, N. and Pope, C. (1995) Rigour and qualitative research. *British Medical Journal*, **311**, 109–112

Mercer, G., Long, A. F. and Smith, I. J. (1995) Researching and evaluating complementary therapies: the state of the debate. Leeds: Collaborating Centre for HSR, Nuffield Institute for Health

Patel, M. S. (1987) Problems in the evaluation of alternative medicine. *Social Science Medicine*, **25**, 669–678

Ross, O. B. Jr and Charlotte, N. C. (1951) Use of controls in medical research. *Journal of the American Medical Association*, **145**, 72–75

Sackett, D. L., Haynes, R. B., Guyatt, G. H. and Tugwell, P. (1991) *Clinical Epidemiology: a Basic Science for Clinical Medicine*, 2nd edn. Boston: Little, Brown and Company

Schlesselman, J. J. (1982) *Case-Control Studies*. New York: Oxford University Press, pp. 680–682

Sheldon, T. A. (1994) Please bypass the PORT. *British Medical Journal*, **309**, 142–143

Vickers, A. (1995) Critical appraisal: how to read a clinical research paper. *Complementary Therapy and Medicine*, **3**, 158–166

Chapter 3

The importance of the placebo effect: a proposal for further research

Jos Kleijnen and Anton J. M. de Craen

Introduction

There is increasing interest in different aspects of the placebo effect. In 1995 there were at least two occasions where a group of scientists met to discuss future research into the placebo effect. These were meetings organized by the Cochrane Collaboration.

Contributors to the Cochrane Collaboration in many countries and specialities are now preparing and maintaining systematic reviews of randomized controlled trials, and reviews of other evidence when appropriate. This international endeavour aims to ensure that, in due course, all areas of health care which have been evaluated using randomized controlled trials will be covered. The reviews prepared and maintained by the Collaboration are disseminated using electronic media through the Cochrane Database of Systematic Reviews.

During the mentioned meetings, topics were addressed that deserved attention in future research. Among these topics were the following:

- systematic exploration and classification of (old) literature
- definition of placebo and placebo response
- what are 'risk-factors' for a placebo response
- mechanisms of action
- unconscious people
- quantification of non-specific effects
- rehabilitation of public image of placebo
- 3-arm trials ('untreated'–placebo–verum)
- 4-arm trials (to test interaction)
- treatment preferences versus randomization
- making use of findings in the psychological, sociological and anthropological literature
- education of doctors

- nocebo effect
- ethical problems when doing research with placebo effects.

Research of the placebo effect

The previous list shows that the subject of placebo research is still very alive. After much attention was paid to this topic in the 1950s and early 1960s interest declined until revival in the 1990s. A number of medical journals have recently published articles discussing the placebo effect in pain treatment and research (Turner *et al.*, 1994), use of placebo controls in clinical trials (Clark and Leaverton, 1994; Rothman and Michels, 1994; Streiner, 1995), misconception of true and perceived placebo effect (Ernst and Resch, 1995), inertness of placebos (Golomb, 1995), efficacy of placebo treatment in patients with amenorrhoea (Crosignani *et al.*, 1994), hypertension (Staessen *et al.*, 1994), varicose veins (Saradeth, Resch and Ernst, 1994), and depression (Brown, 1994). One journal even dedicated a series of seven articles to the subject (Bignall, 1994). In the early years, research into this topic probably did not provide the expected answers. For example, the hypothesis that placebo responders could be identified according to certain psychological characteristics could not be substantiated. In the early 1970s, after Nixon's journey to China, interest in acupuncture increased. Parallel to this, other forms of complementary medicine, including herbal medicine and orthomolecular medicine, became more popular. Many patients and doctors became attracted by a broader view on disease, health and healing: holistic medicine. The recent revival of interest in the placebo effect has certainly been influenced by these developments. This is the case for the use of the placebo effect in daily practice, but also for its role in efficacy research by means of randomized, double-blind clinical trials. Mainstream medicine made justifiable demands concerning the evaluation of the efficacy and effectiveness of complementary medicine.

However, in the process of providing this information about efficacy, many problems arose. Concepts, principles, and philosophies of aetiology, diagnosis, therapy and desired outcomes were different for mainstream and complementary medicine. This of course had consequences for the methodology of research. Even factors which appeared to be simple at first glance, like agreement about a definition of the placebo effect, turned out to be very complex, because of incompatibility of the concepts of different kinds of medicine.

The role of placebo and placebo effects in efficacy research

For many years it has been acknowledged that extraneous factors may considerably influence the size of a therapeutic effect. These extraneous factors, which include placebos, are widely recognized in medicine, but have generally been regarded as a nuisance variable in research. In order to control for these effects in pharmacological research, the randomized, double-blind, placebo-controlled methodology has been developed. The active substance of the medication is assumed to account for the observed difference between the verum and placebo group. This observed difference is usually referred to as the specific effect.

Various systematic reviews on the efficacy of complementary medicine were carried out by one of the authors (ter Riet, Kleijnen and Knipschild, 1990; Kleijnen, Knipschild and ter Riet, 1991; Kleijnen and Knipschild, 1992; Kleijnen, 1994). Corresponding with persons within the field of complementary medicine gave rise to the idea that therapeutic efficacy as measured with the above mentioned specific effect, can only be adequately measured if the atmosphere, the context and the setting of the trial are the same as in clinical practice. There could be interaction between these context variables (we will call them extraneous or non-specific factors), and the specific treatment, e.g. a pharmacological intervention if the specific effect of a medication is modified by the setting of the trial. The effect of a hypotensive drug relative to placebo might be different if both drug and placebo are given in neutral circumstances as opposed to positive circumstances. This example is extensively discussed at the end of this chapter.

There might be a number of parameters that can influence the specific effect of a medication. One frequently cited example is the perceptual characteristic of the medication itself, e.g. colour, size, shape and taste. The following examples illustrate that colour of medication can modify a specific effect of medication. Cattaneo, Lucchetti and Filippuci (1970) administered orange and blue placebos to 120 inpatients awaiting minor surgery, while it was suggested that they were receiving tranquillizers. In this double-blind cross-over study they showed that 26 of 42 men (62%) preferred orange capsules whereas 33 of 54 women (61%) preferred blue capsules.

In another cross-over study, Schapira *et al.* (1970) randomized 48 patients with anxiety symptoms to oxazepam administered in three different colours. Every patient received one week's treatment with each colour. Although statistical significance was not reached, anxiety symptoms were most improved with green and depressive symptoms responded best to yellow.

In a single-blind experiment demonstrating the effect of placebo administration, Blackwell, Bloomfield and Buncher (1972) asked 100 medical students to participate in an experiment in which they would either receive a sedative or stimulant drug. The 56 students who volunteered received either a blue or pink placebo. Drug-associated changes were reported by 30%. Subjects on blue capsules felt less alert (66%), compared with subjects on pink capsules (26%). Furthermore, subjects on blue capsules felt more drowsy (72%), compared with subjects on pink capsules (37%).

Colour of medication is, of course, not the only perceptual characteristic of medication that may influence patients' drug responses. Size of medication and preparation form are other factors that may affect the therapeutic outcome. Buckalew and Coffield (1982) found that capsules were perceived stronger compared with tablets and larger size medication was perceived more potent compared with smaller sizes. Similarly, in a clinical trial comparing chlordiazepoxide capsules with tablets, Hussain (1972) concluded that in the treatment of anxiety the overall response was better when patients were treated with capsules compared with tablets.

The balanced placebo design

In order to investigate possible interaction between specific and non-specific factors, a model design was developed: the balanced placebo design. The model is a factorial design, consisting of a pharmaco-logical intervention (the administration of medication or placebo) and a non-pharmacological intervention (e.g. a positive attitude towards the expected therapeutic effect or a neutral attitude towards the expected therapeutic effect). The hypothesis is that the difference in response between the placebo and verum group (i.e. the specific effect) could be small if the groups are treated in a supportive atmosphere. If the placebo and verum groups were treated in a neutral environment, the specific effect could be larger. This would indicate that the effect size depends on the atmosphere of the trial.

In a recent publication we reviewed 10 studies according to the balanced placebo design. All trials demonstrated a significant influence of a non-specific intervention on the magnitude of the specific effect (Kleijnen et al., 1994). For example, Bergmann et al. (1994) tried to determine whether informed consent modifies the analgesic effect of naproxen and placebo in a randomized, double-blind, cross-over trial. One group received the two treatments uninformed (25 patients) and the other group was asked informed consent and given the two treatments (18 patients, six refused to consent). Pain was assessed on visual analogue scales 30, 60, 120 and 180 minutes after intake of the treatment. The difference in analgesic activity between naproxen and placebo was higher in the uninformed patients: the specific effect was decreased after giving information.

Levine and Gordon (1984), in a randomized, double-blind trial, tested the effects of naloxone or naloxone vehicle in patients who underwent surgery for impacted third molars. The substances were given by one of three methods: by a person at the patient's bedside (open infusion); by a person in an adjacent room (hidden infusion); or by the preprogrammed infusion pump. The effect of the intervention was measured as the change in pain 50 minutes after administration. In the open and hidden infusion groups the naloxone groups experienced more pain than the 'vehicle' groups, but in the machine infusion group the patients who received vehicle experienced more pain than those who were given naloxone. The measured specific effect turned from positive to negative.

Finally, in an experiment to explore interaction between the effect of medication and the effect of the doctor's verbal attitude, Uhlenhuth *et al.* (1966) found that in one clinic the expected drug-placebo difference was apparent, but in the two other participating clinics no such difference existed. They explained this difference by variable clinic features, rather than a non-existing interaction. The difference in response between the control and experimental group was smaller if both groups were treated in a supportive atmosphere, than if both groups were treated in a neutral environment. The 10 studies that were discussed in the review all demonstrated a possible interaction between non-specific and specific intervention. Most studies, however, were considered of average to poor quality.

If interaction were demonstrated in well-performed trials, this could have implications for future randomized controlled trials and may limit the external validity of those conducted previously. It should initiate the development of guidelines for clinical trial settings and therewith improve the methodology of randomized controlled trials. Thus, it might contribute to better efficacy of existing treatments because they may then be carried out in optimal circumstances.

The role of placebo and placebo effects in daily practice

Placebos in clinical trials are given with a different goal than in medical practice. In medical practice a placebo is given with the expectation that, in addition to specific treatment effects, the patient will benefit from the non-specific effects of the placebo. Placebo effects in medical practice should thus be maximized. In clinical trials one is interested in the size of specific effects. In clinical trials placebos are used to distinguish a true pharmacological effect from a non-specific treatment effect and the natural course of disease in that patient. If, in clinical trials, placebo effects are minimized, there is more therapeutic space for the specific effect. For example, if 80% of an improvement is due to placebo effects, only the remaining 20% is available to demonstrate a specific effect. Consequently, in clinical trials, specific effects can be measured more efficiently if placebo effects are small. This results, however, in differences in the treatment settings between medical practice and clinical trials.

In any medical intervention there are placebo effects to some degree. During the meeting between doctors and patients several factors play a role such as the labelling of the therapist by the patient, the credibility of the therapeutic setting, the credibility of the medicine *per se* (size, shape, colour, taste), etc.

The traditional division of the healing process in three parts (effects of self-healing properties of the human body, non-specific effects and specific effects) is of course artificial. As we have shown, it is likely that non-specific factors, such as the doctor's white coat, the colour of medication, informed consent or doctor's and patient's expectancy interact with specific factors. In other words, the size of the specific effect might depend on the circumstances in which the medication is given. Therefore it is very important to know whether and to what extent such interactions take place, so that they can be optimized and used for the benefit of the patient.

Future research

Considering the role of placebo effects in daily practice and in clinical research, we conclude that this topic should clearly be investigated further. In this paragraph we present our plans to assess whether this type of interaction occurs in double-blind, randomized clinical trials. We intend to examine three models, all consisting of one specific intervention (administration of medication) and at least one non-specific intervention. The models will comprise the following: the influence of timing of a questionnaire administration on the effect of bronchodiluent medication or placebo in preoperative pulmonary screening; the effect of positive information on the analgesic activity of a non-steroidal anti-inflammatory drug or placebo in chronic pain patients; the influence of verbal instruction on blood pressure in healthy volunteers after a hypotensive medication or placebo. Below we present one of these trials in detail.

The influence of verbal instructions on blood pressure in healthy volunteers after captopril or placebo

Background

In 1954 Shapiro and co-workers reported a difference in blood pressure response when the same medication was used by an 'enthusiastic' doctor compared with a 'non-enthusiastic' doctor. A similar response has recently been reported by Amigo *et al.* (1993). They demonstrated that orally delivered instructions can modify the intensity and direction of blood pressure measurements. More specifically, normotensive volunteers showed an increase in systolic blood pressure, after they were told that they could expect an increase. Additionally, telling the group they could expect a decrease, induced in fact a decrease in systolic blood pressure.

Goal

This trial is designed to assess the effect of a single dose, oral captopril versus placebo, in healthy volunteers in three different circumstances. Variation in circumstances will be accomplished by randomizing subjects to no information regarding the expected direction of the effect, a mildly positive indication, and an extremely positive indication including the mentioning of possible dizziness.

Subjects

Subjects included in the study will be healthy normotensive volunteers, aged 18–30 years. The following inclusion criterion will be used: body mass index (BMI) between 20 and 30 kg/m^2. The following exclusion criteria will be used: diastolic blood pressure at baseline more than 90 mmHg or systolic blood pressure more than 140 mmHg, current use of medication (except oral contraceptives), possibility of pregnancy.

Interventions

The interventions will be the administration of 50 mg captopril or placebo. Medication distribution will be randomized and double-blind. The non-specific intervention will be that the subject will be told nothing about the expected action, that the expected effect will be a decrease in blood pressure, or that the expected effect can be a rather large decrease in blood pressure and that if they start to feel dizzy, they should report this.

Measurements
After informed consent has been obtained, three baseline blood pressure measurements will be done with one minute intervals using a standard blood pressure apparatus. The mean of the three measurements will be taken as baseline blood pressure. Then the baseline characteristics will be recorded and the randomization carried out. Baseline measurements include sex, date of birth, height, weight, BMI. Automatic blood pressure recordings will be performed for 45 minutes with intervals of 5 minutes after the start of the study medication.

Analysis
The analysis will be as follows: the primary outcome variable will be the difference between the blood pressure after 45 minutes and baseline blood pressure measurement. Some people will react on placebo, some more and some less on captopril. The observed difference between captopril and placebo will be compared between the three groups (neutral attitude, slightly positive and very positive). In this way variation in the specific effect under different circumstances can be shown. But also interaction can be demonstrated. Some people respond on captopril, some on the non-specific intervention, some on both, and maybe some on neither. The part of the population which responds on both the specific and non-specific intervention represents interaction. The effect of the non-specific intervention can be measured by comparing the results in the placebo groups. Interaction is represented by the difference in specific effects, assuming that the susceptibility for the specific intervention is equal for the active groups. Three groups with increasing suggestive information have been chosen because of the possibility of detecting a dose-response curve.

Sample size
It is anticipated that 400 patients will be included. Because the groups should be comparable at baseline and it should be possible to detect small differences, large groups are considered necessary. In the blood pressure trial, the difference between captopril and placebo in the no-information group is expected to be 8 mmHg for systolic blood pressure (large because of minimal placebo response), the expected difference in the minimal information group is 6 mmHg, and the expected difference in the extensive information group is 4 mmHg. The pooled variance estimates is 4.5 mmHg. Using an alpha of 0.05 and a beta of 0.05 this results in a sample size of 400 patients.

Ethical issues in the use and research of placebo and placebo effects

Ethical issues in the use and research of placebo and placebo effects are increasingly important. Many of the studies of the placebo effect performed in the 1950s would be considered unethical nowadays. Asking informed consent for clinical research, nowadays obligatory in many countries, makes certain studies into the placebo effect impossible. For example, telling people that they will be randomized into either an active or a placebo group, but not telling them that they will also be randomized into a positive treatment environment or a neutral one may be considered unethical by some people and some ethical committees. This would make research into this topic impossible, with the consequence that humans will never be able to profit from the knowledge which may be gained from such harmless research. Another often heard criticism is the contrast between strict control of procedures and adherence to ethical norms for clinical research, but virtually no control of similar issues in daily practice. Does every patient in daily practice get such extensive information about all relevant aspects of possible treatment options? The existence of this double standard is only rarely pointed out, and a broader discussion about this topic, by all sections of our community including consumers/patients, doctors, lawyers, politicians and other participants, is clearly warranted.

Conclusion

If interaction is demonstrated, the logical consequence will be that the implicit additive model of the randomized clinical trial is too simple in some if not most occasions. In future studies, non-specific factors which strongly interact with specific treatments must be identified and accounted for. The characteristics of the non-specific effect that define the interaction effects should be identified. For all interventions optimal circumstances in which a maximal treatment effect can be obtained should be assessed. In addition, the circumstances under which the non-specific factors interact should be investigated. Furthermore, the present model on which the randomized clinical trial is based, can then be revised. A more elaborate research methodology needs to be developed taking into account the effect modifiers. We hope that this example will stimulate other researchers to start up similar projects. We feel that there is a need for several investigations to demonstrate that this is an important topic. Once there is general agreement that this is indeed the case, a major research effort is necessary to identify the most important non-specific factors, to uncover the mechanisms of action and to assess the methodological implications and the implications for medical practice.

References

Amigo, I., Cuesta, V., Fernandez, A. and Gonzalez, A. (1993) The effect of verbal instructions on blood pressure measurement. *Journal of Hypertension*, **11**, 293–296

Bergmann, J. F., Chassany, O., Gandiol, J., Deblois, P., Kanis, J. A., Segrestaa, J. M. *et al.* (1994) A randomised clinical trial of the effect of informed consent on the analgesic activity of placebo and naproxen in cancer pain. *Clinical Trials and Meta-Analysis*, **29**, 41–47

Bignall, J. (1994) Science of placebos. *Lancet*, **ii**, 904

Blackwell, B., Bloomfield, S. S. and Buncher, C. R. (1972) Demonstration to medical students of placebo responses and non-drug factors. *Lancet*, 10 June, 1279–1282

Brown, W. A. (1994) Placebo as treatment for depression. *Neuropsychopharmacology*, **10**, 265–269

Buckalew, L. W. and Coffield, K. E. (1982) An investigation of drug expectancy as a function of capsule color and size and preparation form. *Journal of Clinical Psychopharmacology*, **2**, 245–248

Cattaneo, A. D., Lucchelli, P. E. and Filippuci, G. (1970) Sedative effects of placebo treatment. *European Journal of Clinical Pharmacology*, **3**, 43–45

Clark, P. I. and Leaverton, P. E. (1994) Scientific and ethical issues in the use of placebo controls in clinical trials. *Annual Review of Public Health*, **15**, 19–38

Crosignani, P. G., Mattei, A. M., Maggioni, P., Testa, G. and Negri, E. (1994) Efficacy of placebo in the treatment of patients with amenorrhea. *Gynecology and Obstetric Investigation*, **37**, 183–184

Ernst, E. and Resch, K. L. (1995) Concept of true and perceived placebo effects. *British Medical Journal*, **311**, 551–553

Golomb, B. A. (1995) Paradox of placebo effect. *Nature*, **375**, 530

Hussain, M. Z. (1972) Effect of shape of medication in treatment of anxiety states. *British Journal of Psychiatry*, **120**, 507–509

Kleijnen, J. (1994) (Editorial) Evening primrose oil. Currently used in many indications with little justification. *British Medical Journal*, **309**, 824–825

Kleijnen, J., Knipschild, P. and ter Riet, G. (1991) Clinical trials of homoeopathy. *British Medical Journal*, **302**, 316–323

Kleijnen, J. and Knipschild, P. (1992) Ginkgo biloba. *Lancet*, **340**, 1136–1139

Kleijnen, J., de-Craen, A. J. M., van Everdingen, J. and Krol, L. (1994) Placebo effect in double blind clinical trials: a review of interactions with medications. *Lancet*, **ii**, 1347–1349

Levine, J. D. and Gordon, N. C. (1984) Influence of the method of drug administration on analgesic response. *Nature*, **312**, 755–756

Rothman, K. J. and Michels, K. B. (1994) The continuing unethical use of placebo controls. *New England Journal of Medicine*, **331**, 394–398

Saradeth, T., Resch, K. L. and Ernst, E. (1994) Placebo treatment for varicosity: don't eat it, rub it. *Phlebology*, **9**, 63–66

Schapira, K., McClelland, H. A., Griffiths, M. R. and Newell, D. J. (1970) Study on the effects of tablet colour in the treatment of anxiety states. *British Medical Journal*, **2**, 23 May, 446–449

Shapiro, A. P., Myers, T., Reiser, M. F. and Feris, E. B. (1954) Comparison of blood pressure response to veriloid and to the doctor. *Psychosomatic Medicine*, **16**, 478–488

Staessen, J. A., Thÿs, L., Clement, D., Davidson, C., Fagard, R., Lehtonen, A. *et al.* (1994) Ambulatory pressure decreases on long-term placebo treatment in older patients with isolated systolic hypertension. *Journal of Hypertension*, **12**, 1035–1039

Streiner, D. L. (1995) The ethics of placebo-controlled trials. *Canadian Journal of Psychiatry*, **40**: 165–166

ter Riet, G., Kleijnen, J. and Knipschild, P. (1990) Acupuncture and chronic pain. A criteria-based meta-analysis. *Journal of Clinical Epidemiology*, **43**, 1191–1199

Turner, J. A., Deyo, R. A., Loeser, J. D., Von Korff, M. and Fordyce, W. E. (1994) The importance of placebo effects in pain treatment and research. *Journal of the American Medical Association*, **271**, 1609–1614

Uhlenhuth, E. H., Rickels, K., Fisher, S., Park, L. C., Lipman, R. S. and Mock, J. (1966) Drug, doctor's verbal attitude and clinic setting in the symptomatic response to pharmacotherapy. *Psychopharmacologia*, **9**, 392–418

Chapter 4

Complementary medicine: efficacy beyond the placebo effect

Ted J. Kaptchuk, Roger A. Edwards and David M. Eisenberg

Introduction: three theoretical perspectives on the question

One of the most frequently asked questions concerning complementary and alternative medicine therapies is whether they are anything more than placebo effects. This question could be restated as: are any *positive effects* produced by an unconventional medical intervention greater than the effects of a sham intervention in a randomized clinical trial? This chapter discusses this question in relation to complementary and alternative medicine using chiropractic, acupuncture and homoeopathy as specific examples.

The question whether an intervention is more effective than a 'placebo' was asked only a few times in the medical literature before World War II (Gold, Kwit and Otto, 1937; Evan and Hoyle, 1933). It became a common question with the systematic introduction of the randomized clinical trial after World War II (Lilienfeld, 1982). It was not until the 1960s, after the political repercussions of the phocomelia produced by thalidomide, that the comparison of an intervention with a placebo became the pre-eminent question for biomedicine and governmental regulatory agencies.

Before World War II, clinical outcomes were all that mattered in demonstrating effectiveness. Placebo 'controls' came to be considered essential only when it became obvious that non-specific effects were ubiquitous in early clinical experiments. Placebo controls assured that efficacy was due to the 'active' intervention (the dependent variable) and not any non-specific effects. The judgement of efficacy was no longer demonstrable clinical effectiveness but, rather, whether any observable effects adhered to a strict biomedical view of what is important. Efficacy should imitate what Hogben and Sim (1953) called 'a specific stimulus-response nexus', i.e. there must be a mechanical cause and effect relationship between isolated verum intervention and a specific biological/physiological outcome (Lyon, 1990). The question of efficacy had evolved from demonstrable clinical outcomes and gradually became an issue of a demarcation defined by a sham intervention in a clinical trial. This chapter approaches the question of whether efficacy in complementary and alternative medicine is more than the sham intervention of a randomized clinical trial from three distinct theoretical perspectives and then discusses an emerging fourth perspective.

Fastidious efficacy

During the early post-World War II history of clinical experimentation, the tools of randomization and blinding created both the new question of 'what is beyond the placebo' and supplied the mechanism for an answer. The word *fastidious* was first applied to this classic type of randomized clinical trial by Feinstein (1985). The fastidious model of efficacy assumes that verum-specific effects (VSE) and non-specific effects (NSE) are separable and that the total outcome effect (TOE) 'is equal to its active effect plus its placebo effect' (Beecher, 1955). This addition/subtraction approach towards the placebo could be summarized by the following equations:

$$VSE = TOE - NSE$$
$$TOE = VSE + NSE$$
$$NSE = TOE - VSE$$

Non-specific effects are intentionally diminished in placebo controlled clinical trials, if ethically possible, in order that the specific effect can be more efficiently observed. As much as possible, all independent variables are equalized or randomly distributed in the contrived environment of an experiment. Expectation, persuasion, anticipation, belief, faith, suggestion, cultural beliefs, patient–doctor relationship dynamics, imagination and conditioning are all reduced by the blinding processes (especially if double blinding is possible). Minimizing the placebo effect also increases (in theory) the difference between total outcome effect and verum-specific effects so that any measurable effect will be statistically more likely to be observable in a relatively small sample. This approach considers non-specific causation inconsequential and ultimately embodies an implicit value judgement that is dismissive of placebo effects (Sullivan, 1993). This approach was reinforced by the regulatory requirement for efficacy in order to obtain government-approved access to consumers. Nonetheless, with the adoption of statistical methods, the fastidious answer to the question 'efficacy beyond the placebo effect' became quantitative, precise and had the objectiveness that a mechanistic-oriented biology requires.

Pragmatic efficacy

The second approach to the question of what may lie beyond the placebo comes from the perspective of *pragmatic* efficacy, a term coined by Schwartz and Lellouch (1967). The pragmatic approach compares two treatments under conditions in which they would be applied in practice. The pragmatic approach is less concerned with mechanism and explanation. Generally, the research is carried out in a normal or optimal environment with an emphasis on acquiring information necessary for making a clinical decision. In terms of placebo, this model of randomized clinical trials usually assumes that various non-specific effects interact among themselves and among any verum-specific effects; and that it is, therefore, difficult to make a clear distinction between verum and placebo. This approach to placebo, which Uhlenhuth *et al.* (1966) called *interactive*, argues that there is persuasive evidence of synergy between verum-specific and non-specific effects which generate a unique total outcome effect. Specifically, Uhlenhuth *et al.* asked whether non-specific effects could change the verum-specific effects to produce a total outcome effect beyond the effect size of a single fastidious randomized clinical trial or collection of such trials. This interpretation perceives the question of effectiveness as dependent on the interaction of the specific and non-specific effects and 'switch(es) (the question) from whether or not an intervention is a placebo, towards the magnitude of the effect' (Gotzsche, 1994). The pragmatic, interactive approach implicitly questions central facets of the fastidious approach including the assumption that the verum-specific and non-specific effects are stable, separable, linear and relatively constant during the duration of the trial (Spilker, 1991). This model blurs the distinction between verum-specific and non-specific effects and, therefore, implicitly questions the practicality of the question 'what is beyond the placebo effect'. A pragmatic perspective provides less scientifically useful information but potentially provides more clinically relevant information. The growth of the outcomes research is consistent with this pragmatic efficacy construct. From this perspective, 'efficacy beyond the placebo' becomes an inherently unanswerable question.

Performative efficacy

A third approach to this question is what Tambiah (1990) calls *performative* efficacy. This approach is cultural, anthropological, and accepts symbols, belief, suggestion, expectation and persuasion as central to illness and health. This approach avoids reliance on objectivity, controls, and measurement and has no generalization and replicability. Instead, it examines healing as symbolic words and dramatic behaviours that persuasively generate what Csordas (1983) has called 'a predisposition to heal', an experience of empowerment, and concrete perceptions of transformation. These effects are not necessarily possible without the full commitment of the belief, imagination and the will of a participant. This approach has more to do with religion than science and raises the question of who decides what is a sham. Performative efficacy is grounded in the language of solidarity, holism, and unity; and it is immune to the distancing and neutrality requirement of randomization, blinding and *p* values. It generates a clear answer concerning what self-selected, biased and individual people think is 'beyond sham healing'. This approach responds to the question of 'efficacy beyond the placebo effect' by turning it on its head. It asks, instead, who decides whether a therapy is merely sham or more than sham? The performative efficacy approach can only be documented in anthropological studies (qualitative research on performative efficacy) and patient satisfaction surveys (qualitative and quantitative research on performative efficacy) which generally rely on primarily subjective outcomes. This perspective points to the possibility that one answer to the question, what is beyond a sham intervention, is defined by the eyes of the beholder, who may or may not recognize the scientific method as the final arbitrator.

Fastidious efficacy and complementary medicine

The evidence: chiropractic and manipulation versus sham

The earliest attempts to evaluate fastidiously spinal manipulative therapy with a randomized clinical trial began in 1974 at the Welsh National School of Medicine (Glover, Morris and Kholsa, 1974). Since then, there have been at least 25 randomized clinical trials for spinal manipulative therapy (Skellele *et al.*, 1992) and low back pain, nine of which compared spinal manipulative therapy to a sham intervention. This chapter adopts the common practice of discussing all spinal manipulative therapy as if it were equivalent to chiropractic manipulation, although we recognize that this approach can lead to major confounding issues (Assendelft *et al.*, 1992). Of the nine fastidious trials, three show no difference between manipulation and a sham (Sims-Williams *et al.*, 1979; Godfrey, Morgan and Schatzher, 1984; Gibson *et al.*, 1985), two are positive for manipulation (Bergquist-Ullman and Larsson, 1977; Waagen *et al.*, 1986), one is clearly positive for manipulation plus injected drug (Ongley *et al.*,

1987) and, depending on how one identifies significant outcomes measures (especially in terms of the time variable), three trials could be construed as showing some benefit for manipulation over sham during some course of the complaint (Glover, Morris and Kholsa, 1974; Sims-Williams *et al.*, 1978; Hoehler, Tobis and Buerger, 1981). There are also two randomized clinical trials comparing spinal manipulative therapy to sham in the treatment of hypertension; the 18-week trial showed no difference (Morgan *et al.*, 1985) while the short-term trial of a single treatment was significantly positive for spinal manipulative therapy (Yates, 1988). The great majority of other trials including those for neck and head pain, comparing spinal manipulative therapy to another treatment are a hybrid approach roughly between what this chapter defines as fastidious and pragmatic: while there are two 'true' treatments (like in a pragmatic trial), there is an attempt to keep all other variables (e.g. attention, environment, expectation, therapist attitudes, etc.) equal (like a fastidious trial). These trials have some of the pro and cons of each approach and often methodologically and imprecisely blend both approaches so that it is unclear what they contribute to our question. They reflect an attempt to conform to the fastidious model while simultaneously striving for clinical relevance in the context of the limitations of implementation.

The evidence: homoeopathy versus placebo

Homoeopaths have sought to use comparative clinical trials to demonstrate the effectiveness of their medical system from the onset and often demanded and undertook comparative clinical trials (Kaufman, 1971; Cassedy, 1984; King, 1991); the testing of placebo versus homoeopathic remedy began at the same time as clinical researchers introduced the method in the UK. The famous 1943 mustard gas trials may have had a sham control (*British Homoeopathic Journal*, 1943; Paterson, 1944) and, certainly, by 1954, placebo controlled clinical trials were part of homoeopathic research (Ledermann, 1954). We rely on the much cited meta-analysis performed at the University of Limberg (Kleijnen, Knipschild and ter Riet, 1991) as evidence of fastidious efficacy in homoeopathy. This team reviewed 107 controlled homoeopathy trials (68 of which were randomized), over a wide assortment of clinical issues (including cardiovascular disease – 9, respiratory infections – 19, disease of the GI tract – 7, hay fever – 5, rheumatic disease – 6, trauma and/or pain – 20. Their 'voting meta-analysis' which did not statistically aggregate across trials, showed that 81 trials had positive effects and 24 lacked positive effects. It seems the great majority of these trials were fastidious; the Kleijnen team reported that 'most' of the trials had placebo controls (as opposed to active intervention treatments) but did not cite an exact number. (An earlier more limited meta-analytic review of 40 randomized homoeopathic trials also reported that the great majority of trials (36) were placebo controlled) (Hill and Doyon, 1990). The Kleijnen group paper had an unusual conclusion. They felt that the evidence presented in their review 'would probably be sufficient for establishing homoeopathy as a regular treatment for certain indications' but, presumably because there is no 'plausible mechanism of action', they called for 'a few well performed controlled trials in humans with large numbers of participants under rigorous double-blind conditions'. The Hill and Doyon (1990) meta-analysis which aggregated statistical outcomes did not find evidence for homoeopathy's efficacy.

The evidence: acupuncture versus sham

Since 1974, with the publication of two trials from the University of Manitoba (Man and Baragar, 1974; Anderson, Jamieson and Man, 1974), both of which compared acupuncture with sham acupuncture for pain, this East Asian medical practice has been the subject of a large number of randomized clinical trials. Eisenberg (1995), in an ongoing survey of randomized clinical trials of acupuncture, has identified 228 clinical trials concerning acupuncture performed over a wide range of clinical concerns including 137 for pain; 21 for nausea; 20 in ophthalmology and otolaryngology; 19 for substance abuse; 15 for cerebrovascular illnesses; seven for neurological problems; five for gynaecological complaints and four for gastrointestinal problems. The randomized clinical trials for pain included 45 for chronic, 19 for musculoskeletal, 18 for headache, 14 for low back, 12 for osteo-arthritis, 11 for dental, seven for experimentally-induced, five for shoulder, three for cervical and three for facial pain. Since chronic pain is the single most studied area of possible acupuncture efficacy, it serves as a benchmark for discussion of the acupuncture versus sham question. Again, we will rely on two previously published meta-analyses of acupuncture for chronic pain that drew similar conclusions on acupuncture's efficacy beyond placebo (but had different conclusions on the likelihood of acupuncture's efficacy in general).

A team from the Institut Universitaire de Médecine Sociale et Préventive in Lausanne pooled 14 randomized clinical trials of acupuncture for pain and analysed them in a variety of subgroups (e.g. for all pain, for low back pain, for head/neck pain, acupuncture versus conventional treatment for head/neck pain, larger trials versus smaller trials, partially blind versus no blinding, Chinese or acupuncture journal versus mainstream medical journal, etc.) (Patel *et al.*, 1989). They believed that methodological shortcomings precluded conclusive results but that, overall, most results 'apparently favoured acupuncture' and therefore the meta-analysis was generally positive towards acupuncture's efficacy. However, for the subgroup of six trials that compared acupuncture with sham, no significant differences were obtained.

In the following year, ter Riet, Kleijnen and Knipschild, (1990) (the same Limberg team who wrote the homoeopathy paper), published a meta-analysis of 51 controlled clinical studies on the effectiveness of acupuncture in chronic pain. Performing a 'voting' meta-analysis they found 24 studies had significant positive results and 27 studies had negative outcomes. Because the results were 'highly contradictory', their opinion was that acupuncture's efficacy remained 'doubtful'. Ter Riet, Kleijnen and Knipschild (1990) also performed a separate subgroup analysis for studies employing sham procedures which totalled 32 studies of which 17 were negative and 15 positive. Like the Patel subgroup, the results of acupuncture versus sham for chronic pain were inconclusive, doubtful or too contradictory for a clear interpretation.

Complementary and alternative medicine versus sham from the fastidious efficacy perspective: some observations

Generally speaking, the evidence from a large number of complementary and alternative medicine trials suggests that the answer to the question of efficacy beyond placebo is unknown from the fastidious efficacy perspective. However, all studies have methodological limitations to varying degrees that might explain these equivocal or contradictory findings. The concept of fastidious efficacy is based on the extrapolation of laboratory experiments to ill human beings. In the process of attempting to recreate laboratory conditions in human beings in a democratic society, many practical implementation and conceptual problems are evident: sufficient sample size; time to complete; generalization – external validity – since trials often exclude various subgroups of patients for a range of reasons, such as age, severity, comorbidities, childbearing potential; difficulty of enrolment; patient consent and recruitment; choice of measurable endpoints versus clinically meaningful endpoints or patient-relevant endpoints; specific challenges of implementing proper blinding and randomization; cost; difficulties with assumptions underlying statistics and statistical analyses such as choice of appropriate statistical procedure and hypothesis testing. (Louis and Shapiro, 1983; Pocock, 1985; Greenfield, 1989; Reilly and Findley, 1989; Spilker, 1991;

Rogers, 1994; Rosner, 1995). These limitations apply to all trials whether complementary and alternative medicine or conventional.

The difficulties are evident in the review by Williamson, Goldschmidt and Colton (1986) of the conventional medical literature. 'Serious, widespread problems exist in the published clinical literature' and 'only 6% of the trials met the minimum design and statistical criteria established by the authors of the 12 methodological reviews' (Ottenbacher, 1992). All these constraints may contribute to the lack of clarity present in the fastidious approach to efficacy. But it can readily be observed that many conventional therapies demonstrate efficacy despite these limitations.

In terms of complementary and alternative medicine, these potential problems may be compounded (Anthony, 1993). It is unclear whether most of the fastidious trials have adequate knowledge concerning complementary and alternative medicine. Until very recently, it was not easy for serious academic researchers to collaborate with 'fringe' alternative healers. The acupuncture or spinal manipulative therapy treatments in many of the trials are of insufficient 'dose' for there to be a reasonable expectation of success. In most complementary and alternative medicine trials, the training and qualifications of the providers seems undetermined or inadequate. Few trials attempted to take into consideration the conceptual and therapeutical models of the system or stratify for distinct complementary and alternative medicine diagnoses that do not correspond to biomedical nosology. Even fewer trials tried to measure for relative suitability for complementary medicine treatment. What is an appropriate sham in acupuncture is still being debated (Lewith and Machin, 1983; Vincent and Lewith, 1995). External validity is especially problematic in these fastidious complementary and alternative medicine trials (Vickers, 1995). For example, only 14 of the homoeopathic trials used the most common forms of individual homoeopathy (rhetorically referred to as classical). Few of the acupuncture trials used the most common approaches used in modern China and the contemporary West (usually referred to as 'traditional Chinese medicine') and of course, only a handful of the spinal manipulative therapy trials were chiropractic (Assendelft et al., 1992). Money for large scale trials in complementary and alternative medicine has been especially scarce so that inadequate sample sizes make statistically significant results more difficult to obtain.

A second general observation of the fastidious evidence for complementary medicine is that the complaints and illnesses that are most often the subject of complementary and alternative medicine research and practice are the most difficult to adapt to a fastidious model. Fastidious trials are best performed with clear entry and outcome measures and diseases that conform to clinico-anatomical conceptions and have 'ontological self-sufficiency' (Tauber, 1994). The method performs best with hard and clear data. Peculiarly, complementary and alternative medicine research and practice most often deals with complaints that are deeply connected to changes in subjective awareness, perception and self-monitoring. The foundations of the complementary and alternative medicine industry which are reflected in the randomized clinical trial literature seem to have four main sources: illnesses that have highly subjective components (e.g. chronic pain, low back pain, insomnia, headache, anxiety and allergies); chronic illnesses with fluctuating courses that are also highly sensitive to subjective states (e.g. arthritis and asthma); somatizing disorders due to highly vigilant monitoring of normal bodily sensations (e.g. some forms of chronic fatigue, hypoglycae-mia); and minor self-limiting ailments (e.g. colds and minor trauma). It is precisely these areas that need the biggest sample sizes and provide the most muddled and imprecise measurements. Reproduci-bility and generalization also become more tenuous. (Patients with cancer or HIV infection are frequent users of complementary and alternative medicine therapies but they represent a tiny proportion of all users and randomized clinical trials (Eisenberg et al., 1993).)

There is a third observation that could be made after reading the meta-analytic review and health policy literature. It may be that for certain problems where conventional medicine is impoverished for an adequate response (e.g. low back pain) the criteria for scientific evaluation do not have to demonstrate superiority over sham to receive the positive support from scientific evaluations or government approval. For example, the meta-analytic analyses for manipulation and low back pain aggregate manipulation versus sham trials, manipulation versus conventional treatment (in the hybrid fastidious/ pragmatic form) to estimate effect size (e.g. Shekelle et al., 1992) despite the fact that 'manipulation' is not the same in each trial and often not described. Decisions are made based on all the available evidence and evident need for treatment, not merely the evidence from the fastidious efficacy perspective. For example, the US government's Agency for Health Care Policy and Research's (AHCPR) *Clinical Practice Guideline for Acute Low Back Problems in Adults* in December 1994, declared with a level B strength of evidence that 'manipulation can be helpful for patients with acute low back problems without radiculopathy when used within the first month of symptoms' (Bigos et al., 1994).

A fourth observation from this review is that even when 'good' evidence exists with double-blind randomized clinical trials, as is the case in the homoeopathy trials, prior beliefs still affect the evaluation of efficacy beyond placebo. Because the prior belief in homoeopathy of the Limberg team was apparently zero or very low, they concluded that the complementary medicine intervention (homoeopathy) should be tested in placebo-controlled trials more times than would be necessary for a therapy grounded in conventional notions of science. 'Scientific proof' really means replication and convergence of evidence, both empirical and theoretical. Since complementary and alternative medicine is often based on non-conformist medical ideologies, the demand for evidence may be higher and more methodologically rigorous than is usually expected. Therefore, the efficacy beyond placebo question may remain unanswered from the fastidious efficacy perspective for some time.

Pragmatic efficacy

Evidence for the interactive model of placebo

Evidence that non-specific effects have a huge variance and that the verum-specific and non-specific effects interact in dramatic and significant ways has accumulated for decades. Wolf pioneered studies on the relationship of pharmacologically active drugs, suggestion, and conditioning in over 100 experiments on human subjects including one patient with a large gastric fistula, in whom it was possible to observe directly the gastric mucus membrane (Wolf, 1950). In these studies, when the principal subject was told that drug had a certain effect (NSE), various drug effects (VSE) were subjectively and objectively reversed. A significant number of the almost 1000 annotated bibliographic citations on pre-1978 research concerning placebo also demonstrate this proposition; although most studies have serious methodological flaws (Turner, Gallimore and Fox-Henning, 1980). Kleijnen et al. (1994) in an important essay in the 1994 *Lancet* series on placebo, cautiously summarized some of the critical evidence: 'there may ... be interaction between component of treatment ... Specific and non-specific effects are sometimes synergistic, and at other times antagonistic, so that the implicit additive model of the randomized clinical trial is too simple'.

Kleijnen and colleagues mention among other experiments: the study by Uhlenhuth et al. (1966) of the effects of enthusiasm versus a hesitant tone (non-specific effects) on the tranquillizer meprobamate (verum-specific effects); the study by Gracely et al. (1985) documenting provider expectation significantly changing non-specific effects; and the study by Skovlund (1991) where patient knowledge of whether they were likely to receive a real analgesic (i.e. participate in head to head trial) or only possibly receive a real analgesic (i.e. participate in a placebo-controlled trial) changed total outcome effect, non-specific and verum-specific effects. The Kleijnen team's strict and narrow entrance criteria for their study eliminated a huge number of additional studies that also provide evidence for non-specific and verum-specific effects interaction.

The fastidious model's assumption of a stable, separable, linear and relatively constant placebo effect in clinical trials is still an assumption and much contrary evidence exists. 'Subtract the placebo response from the medicine response to obtain a net medicine-induced response ... this commonly used technique probably represents a simplification and rests on several unproven assumptions: (1) part of the medicine response results from a placebo effect, (2) the same amount of a medicine response results from a placebo effect as in the placebo group or placebo phase of a trial, (3) if the same patient has received both medicine and placebo, the baseline and conditions under which they were each taken were the same, (4) the placebo and medicine responses are linear, and (5) the placebo response is relatively constant in magnitude throughout the duration of the trial. The interaction of a trial medicine and placebo, however, is probably complex, and some of these assumptions are probably not valid' (Spilker, 1991).

Spilker's cautions are consistent with the conclusion of White, Tursky and Schwartz (1985) that a 'systems theory perspective' is needed to address the complex interactions of placebo-related phenomena. Such an approach is a 'metatheoretical framework for integrating biological, psychological, and social influences on health and illness ... composed of subsystems that interact at all levels via a complex network of feedback and feed-forward loops ... out of the interaction of the parts, there emerge new properties that are unique to the system or entity as a whole. Emergent properties are more than simple, independent sum of the properties of the part studied in isolation ... emergent phenomena are universal in nature, and occur at all levels of complexity' (White, Turksky and Schwartz, 1985).

Other evidence for interaction not included in the Kleijnen review includes the following examples: the study by Sarles, Camatte and Sahel (1977) where different physicians treating the duodenal ulcer had different outcomes for both verum-specific and non-specific effect; the study by Wolf (1962) where different researchers (non-specific effects) consistently produced either increased or decreased gastric secretions when they gave a placebo (non-specific effects) to patients; the study by Penik and Fisher (1965) where epinephrine (verum-specific effect) was turned into a stimulant or neutral substance depending on expectation (non-specific effect); the study by Jensen and Karoly (1991) where motivation and expectation changed reaction to a sedative drug; the study by Penick and Hickle (1964) where phenmetrazine only had an effect on food intake if patients were informed (non-specific effect) of the drug's effect (verum-specific effect); the meta-analysis by Hulland Bond (1986) of 'balanced placebo' designed trials showing alcohol consumption and expectancy significantly interacting; the study by Hughes *et al.* (1989) where various forms of instruction (non-specific effect) significantly interacted with nicotine (verum-specific effect) in smoking cessation; and the study by Kirsch and Rosandino (1993) study where caffeine only had a verum-specific effect when non-specific effects were manipulated. This illustrative but not exhaustive list suggests tentative conclusions due to the studies' methodological flaws. Nonetheless, the evidence adds further weight to the argument for an interactive placebo effect rather than an additive one. Therefore, the interactive model argues that the additive model on which the question beyond placebo is based is incomplete and oversimplified. Non-specific effects cannot be linearly extracted from verum-specific effects because such subtraction is not consistent with the decades of evidence and theory to the contrary.

Evidence for a mega-placebo effect

Non-specific effects can be large; the magnitude of these effects is rarely a significant subject in the medical literature since Beecher's original peculiar proto-meta-analysis (1955). Beecher's numbers (35% ± 2%) are routinely accepted and repeated. The literature is mostly concerned with verum-specific effects or the verum-specific plus non-specific effects (i.e. total outcome effect) size. The independent status of non-specific effects tends to be marginalized. One possible component of the pragmatic perspective that needs to be raised, relates to the potential size of the non-specific effects. The general assumption is that verum-specific plus non-specific effects of a proven truly effective treatment (Ttx) is going to be greater than the non-specific effects of a disproven ineffective false treatment (Ftx). The presupposition can be stated as follows:

$$VSE + NSE_{of\ Ttx} > NSE_{of\ Ftx}\ \text{(which, by designation, has no VSE)}$$

The medical literature has not addressed (so far as we can determine; although Klaus Linde [personal communication, 1994] of München and Herman Engelbart [personal communication, 1992] of Amsterdam have verbally expressed it) that it may be possible for the non-specific effects of a false therapy to be greater than the verum-specific and non-specific effects of a true treatment. This possibility can be stated as follows:

$$NSE_{of\ Ftx}(i.e.\ TOE_{of\ Ftx}) > VSE + NSE_{of\ Ttx}(\ i.e.\ TOE_{of\ Ttx})$$

We call this effect a 'mega-placebo' and it raises the possibility that one dimension of efficacy beyond the placebo of a randomized clinical trial is a scientific anomaly. A false 'unscientific' treatment could have a larger total outcome effect in a particular condition than a 'proven scientific' treatment. It may be possible in some conditions that the non-specific effects of a complementary and alternative medicine therapy have a greater total outcome effect than its scientific counterpart. For example, assuming acupuncture has no verum-specific effect, it might still have a non-specific effect (and, therefore, a total outcome effect) greater than non-steroidal anti-inflammatory drugs in chronic pain. One possible answer for what 'lies beyond   the placebo of a randomized clinical trial' is a 'mega-placebo'. This entire discussion creates a genuine conundrum and scientific paradox. We are not arguing that it is true; only that it is possible and needs   to be investigated. Nonetheless, we want to raise its possibility and offer some tentative and flawed evidence for considering its further investigation. A sampling of evidence might include the following.

The early research of Wolf (1950) at Cornell University Medical School has already been mentioned. He was able to have non-specific effects reinforce or totally override the pharmacological actions of a wide variety of drugs (verum-specific effects). In elaborate experiments that traced objective physiology, Wolf used non-specific effects such as suggestion (saying the drug had its opposite effect) or conditioning (by giving a series of the opposite acting drugs first), to counteract completely verum-specific effects. For example, ipeca-cuanha became an anti-emetic and atropine a gastric stimulator. Although these first experiments were on single subjects and had unclear blinding procedures and controls, they remain suggestive that non-specific effects can be greater than verum-specific effects.

The well-known single blind randomized experiment comparing internal mammary artery ligation and sham operation for angina pectoris treated a total of 18 patients – five of whom received sham procedures (Dimond, Kittle and Crockett, 1960). The follow up averaged 4.5 months and of the sham group, two patients had 100% improvement and the other three had 'definite benefit' (between 50 and 90% improvement) on such scales as lessened need for nitroglycerine, tolerance to exercise, and sense of well-being. The genuine surgery group did less well. Although the study had no untreated arm which would allow a clear evaluation of the magnitude of the placebo response, the non-specific effect in this trial was large and had a significant total outcome effect.

Sox, Margulies and Sox (1981) demonstrated that drop-in Veterans Administration clinic patients with chest pain who received diagnostic tests believed that they had better care and recovered quicker than those who had not received tests. Idler and Kasl (1991) in their re-analysis of 4-year follow-up mortality data of 2812 patients concluded that, 'an independent effect . . . of self-evaluation of health status (exists) . . . to predict mortality, above and beyond the contribution to prediction made by indices based on the presence of health problems, physical disability, and biological or life-style risk factors'.

Very recently, the US government's Agency for Health Care Policy and Research's *Clinical Practice Guidelines on Benign Prostatic Hyperplasia: Diagnosis and Treatment* (McConnell *et al.*, 1994) presented a curious anomaly that provides further evidence of a 'mega-placebo'. The pooled aggregate placebo effect in several interventions for benign prostatic hypertrophy (excluding finasteride but including alpha blocker, balloon dilation, transurethral incision of the prostate, transurethral resection of the prostate and open prostatectomy) (i.e. non-specific effect) was greater than the treatment effect of finasteride, which is a proven true treatment. Sham procedures have a greater aggregate total outcome effect than a true drug treatment. This example obviously has the serious flaw that it involves a comparison between different randomized groups and insufficient statistics appear in the text to check some of the discussion. Nonetheless, it is provocative. The non-specific effect (and total outcome effect) of a false intervention seem to be greater than the total outcome effect of a true intervention. This is one outcome that could possibly happen with complementary and alternative medicine treatments that might be observed in a pragmatic randomized clinical trial.

The evidence for complementary and alternative medicine from the pragmatic efficacy approach

The majority of the randomized clinical trials in the area of chiropractic/spinal manipulative therapy and acupuncture are hybrid outcome studies. They compare two types of therapies (e.g. spinal manipulative therapy versus 'back school', acupuncture versus drug) and try to 'equalize' all other variables. They are partly fastidious and partly pragmatic and do not clearly answer the fastidious question nor the pragmatic question. The homoeopathic trials are mostly fastidious; few are pragmatic or hybrid-pragmatic.

Relatively few complementary and alternative medicine pragmatic trials exist where each arm is allowed to work in 'optimal' circumstances with duration, type and frequency of the treatment decided totally at the discretion of the therapist. A pragmatic trial generally allows non-specific effects to interact freely. There are relatively few such trials. The two largest, most well-designed and significant trials in the domains we are considering are both pragmatic trials of spinal manipulative therapy. One is that by Meade *et al.* (1990) and its extended follow up (Meade *et al.*, 1995) in the UK and the other, the study by Koes *et al.* (1992, 1993) in Holland.

The Meade study enrolled 741 patients with low back pain who went either to one of 11 chiropractic offices or 11 matched conventional hospital clinics. Rather than follow up their self-selection choice, these patients were instead randomly assigned to either chiropractic care or conventional care. Only 28% of those who were asked at the chiropractors' offices agreed to randomization, compared with 80% at the hospital sites. This probably removed from the study a disproportionate number of patients who were especially biased favourably towards a positive chiropractic experience, possibly introducing a negative bias towards chiropractic in the study. The conclusions of the investigators were dramatic: 'Chiropractic care was more effective than hospital outpatient management, mainly for patients with chronic or severe back pain. A benefit of about 7% points on the Oswestry (pain disability) scale was seen at two years. The benefit of chiropractic treatment became more evident throughout the follow-up period. Secondary outcomes measures also showed that chiropractic was more beneficial ... For patients with low back pain ... chiropractic almost certainly confers worthwhile, long term benefit in comparison with hospital outpatient management'. The benefit is seen mainly in those with chronic and severe pain'.

The researchers called for chiropractic's inclusion in the British National Health Service. (It should be noted that conventional care in the UK included Maitland (72%) and Cyriax (12%) spinal manipulation therapy, which in the USA would still be alternative.) In the extended follow up which reported on all patients who were followed for 3 years the conclusions were similar: 'according to total Oswestry scores improvement in all patients at three years was about 29% more in those treated by chiropractors than in those treated by the hospitals. The beneficial effect of chiropractic on pain was particularly clear' (Meade, 1995).

This comparative trial and its follow up present clear evidence that, in the UK, chiropractic care is superior than conventional care. This could mean:

$$VSE_{chiropractic} + NSE_{chiropractic} > VSE_{conventional} + NSE_{conventional} \text{ or}$$

$$NSE_{chiropractic} > VSE_{conventional} + NSE_{conventional}$$

(the 'mega-placebo' situation) or

$$NSE_{chiropractic} > NSE_{conventional} \text{ (assuming neither has any VSE).}$$

The pragmatic trial has no way of determining which of these three equations is operational. Some argue that it does not matter. It does say that chiropractic, at this point in the UK, delivers a total outcome effect which is greater than conventional low back care. Its answer to 'beyond the placebo effect' is to disregard the questions and give a pragmatic response designed to make a medical decision. Meade *et al.* (1995) also called for more fastidious studies.

The study by Koes *et al.* (1992, 1993) while not as dramatic shows roughly the same picture. It enrolled 256 patients with non-specific back and neck pain of at least 6 weeks' duration and randomized them to four arms: manual therapy, physiotherapy, general medical care and a placebo treatment of detuned shortwave diathermy. The first three arms were genuinely pragmatic. The results were 'improvement in the main complaint was larger with manipulative therapy (4.5) than with physiotherapy (3.8) after 12 months' follow up (differences 0.9; 95% confidence interval 0.1 to 1.7)' (1992). Placebo treatment and general medicine were clearly inferior to either manipulation or physiotherapy. The trial presented clear evidence that in Holland manipulative therapy is better for back/neck pain. Whether these results were because of verum-specific effects, an amplified non-specific effect or even mega-placebo effects is undetermined. Cleverly, because of the fourth fastidious arm, this pragmatic trial also showed that manipulative therapy was better than a regular (non-amplified?) placebo effect. (Curiously, the placebo had a better outcome than the general medicine arm which may have been because of amplified non-specific effects, mega-placebo effects or even because general medicine in back/neck pain has a negative outcome effect. Interpreting the general medicine and placebo arm is however difficult because of a high number of patients who changed assignments in these two arms.) This study presents clear evidence that manipulation is effective in a pragmatic way in Holland while at the same time showing in a more fastidious manner that it is also better than a normal placebo effect.

Performative efficacy

The question of 'beyond placebo' is integral to the fastidious and current scientific perspective. It is a new question that the biomedical world has only recently adopted and accepted. The public barely understands it. One problem with the question is that it implicitly restricts the meaning of healing to the following: healing is the cause and effect relationship between a specific intervention and defined biological outcome. In fact, ordinary people obtain much more from healers and healing than this definition implies. The general population does not confine their evaluation of whether a treatment is more than a sham to this narrow perspective. 'Beyond placebo effect' may mean it 'works' in the subjective context of their lives.

Performative efficacy in healing

Healing rituals have a performative efficacy that provides a 'pathway of words, feelings, values, expectations . . . which reorder and organize the disease experience' (Klienman, 1973) whether or not any biological efficacy is present. Healing provides 'imaginative possibilities, behavioural options and rhetorical supplies' (Kirmayer, 1993). Behind the emblem of the 'art of medicine' conventional medicine also fosters this aspect of healing which requires trust, commitment, participation and relies on persuasion, expectancy, suggestion, hope and moral authority. In order for this dimension of health care to occur, the medical rituals must be believed in – 'not in the sense that their truth value is certified by logic or argument but in the sense that they are taken into the imagination and lived with, if only for a time' (Kirmayer, 1993). But the randomized clinical trial neglects or more exactly disposes of, through blinding, informed consent and randomization, this dimension of healing. Commitment, connection and 'full subjective participation' are not allowed. Scientific knowledge, at least during a randomized clinical trial, makes an ethical and epistemological assumption that a particular scientific knowledge has a higher value than these subjective dimensions of health care. A blinded, randomized clinical trial is incapable of evaluating whether a particular therapy or type of therapy for a particular condition with this kind of belief committment provides this kind of performative efficacy better than another. (A pragmatic trial probably could assess some, but not all, of these dimensions.)

The complementary and alternative medicine cosmos, empowerment and concern

The complementary and alternative medicine universe is profoundly different from the conventional world. The conventional biomedicine world's scientific language is objective, neutral, analytic, experimental, and distant. While complementary and alternative medicine also shares some of this style of language – there is a 'science' of chiropractic, acupuncture and homoeopathy – something else is going on. The language of complementary and alternative medicine is also framed in terms of solidarity, unity, holism and the sense of encompassing oneness (Tambiah, 1990). The complementary and alternative medicine universe is filled with benign, benevolent, and intentional forces. The *innate intelligence* of chiropractic, the *qi* of acupuncture and the *vital spiritual force* of homoeopathy have persuasive rhetorical effects. Just when a person is debilitated and feels fragile and broken, these alternative medical systems connect a person in a web of words and a dramatic ritual of actions to a persuasive experience of a cosmos concerned with human welfare, intelligent and infinite in resources. Complementary and alternative medicine offers not only treatment for problems but a realignment in relationship to these problems. A 'full participant' in chiropractic, acupuncture, or homoeopathy is having more than their spine adjusted with hands, their meridians opened with acupuncture needles, and their spiritualized life force finally connected to its dematerialized counterpart. Or as Oths (1994) has said about chiropractic: 'in essense, the chiropractor first manipulates a patient's belief structure before manipulating his or her physical structure'. Complementary and alternative medicine provides a renewed context of hope and empowerment.

Complementary and alternative medicine, disease, labelling and connection

Diseases that resist clear labelling and explanation in biomedicine – chronic pain, low back pain, chronic fatigue, arthritis, allergies – are all either easily diagnosed (in chiropractic or acupuncture) or profoundly understood (in homoeopathy). There is little discrepancy between the patient's experience and provider model.

Complementary and alternative medicine also provides significant meaning for an illness. A person's troubles are all situated in a cosmic drama of vital energies that can be nurtured, fostered, and fully embraced. The clinical encounter with a complementary and alternative medicine provider allows for an enlargement of self-identity and personal connection just when sickness threatens to rob a person of their fundamental sense of connectedness.

Complementary and alternative medicine and the perception of transformation

Complementary and alternative medicine also provides tangible perceptions of transformation (Csordas, 1983). The chiropractor will very often produce a very audible 'pop' of the spine during an adjustment. The adjustment itself, because it moves vertebrae beyond their previous range of motion at least momentarily increases mobility and flexibility. The acupuncturist will be able to feel the *qi* and be able to point to at least one of the many signs and symptoms in their domain of concern to indicate that the *qi* has been reactivated. The homoeopath can do it either way: either things get better in some way or there is an exacerbation of symptoms (following Hering's law). Both directions provide evidence that the *vital force* is resonating with the remedy. Finding this kind of evidence to support a perception of metamorphosis in complementary and alternative medicine is relatively easy especially if the patient has an illness with a variable course and highly influenced by subjective monitoring. This kind of inference is even easier in self-limiting illness.

It may even be possible that these performative dimensions change the long-term course of some illnesses through a change in 'somatic mode of attention' (Csordas, 1994). It may be that some of the pragmatic efficacy shown in the Meade study discussed above may have to do with these factors. The 'independent effect' in Idler and Kasl's research (1991) may also reflect these performative dimensions as a baseline regardless of any healing interventions.

Performative efficacy and the randomized controlled trial

Randomization, blinding and informed consent are all attempts to neutralize performative efficacy. They help remove patient 'knowledge', 'commitment' and 'faith'. These endeavours to uncover 'scientific' and biological based 'truths' probably introduce another set of artificial bias and probably hamper certain dimensions of generalization from a randomized clinical trial (Llewellyn-Thomas, 1991). Informed consent itself is a potent non-specific effect (Dahan, 1986; Myers *et al.*, 1987) and changes clinical outcomes. Bergmann's (1994) highly unusual (and ethically problematical study) of giving drug and placebo in both informed and uninformed circumstances showed that informed consent can reverse, in a 'mega-placebo' fashion, verum-specific, non-specific and total outcome effects. Blinding can change verum-specific effects and even prevent their detectability, not to mention modifying non-specific effects (Kirsch and Rosadino, 1993; Kirsch and Weixel, 1988). Preference effects can also be significant (Barry *et al.*, 1995; Wennberg, 1990; Henshaw, 1993). The performative perspective raises the question that the randomized clinical trial may create its own unintended biases and distortions. For example, it is likely that from the perception of the 72% of the patients at the chiropractor's office in Meade's study

(1990) who refused to be randomized, many might think the only 'sham' involved in the chiropractic randomized clinical trial was the trial itself. (Unfortunately, as in most studies, people who refused to be randomized were not followed in the Meade study.)

Performative efficacy: the evidence

One of the ways to obtain a sense of how non-randomized, self-selected, biased and ordinary people subjectively experience complementary and alternative medicine is by patient surveys. Here the evidence for whether people think complementary and alternative medicine is more than a sham is clearly postive.

The largest survey questioning people concerning their satisfaction with 'questionable health treatments' was conducted by Louis Harris and Associates (Harris *et al.*, 1987) in the USA for the Department of Health and Human Services. The figures are impressively in favour of complementary and alternative medicine: eight out of 10 users reported satisfaction (42% were *very satisfied* and another 38% were *somewhat satisfied*).

Patient satisfaction data for acupuncture or homoeopathy seems to vary considerably depending on the population studied; on average it is good and patients perceive these therapies to be effective (Ernst, 1996). For chiropractic in the USA, the evidence repeats the Harris poll. A 1989 survey of 500 randomly selected Connecticut households found that of the 21% of the respondents who had visited chiropractors at least once, 78% felt the treatment was *effective* or *very effective* (Wardwell, 1989); a 1991 telephone interview of 693 households in New Jersey recorded user satisfaction in the 'effectiveness' of their treatment at 88% (23% *satisfied*, 65% *fully satisfied*) (Sawyer and Kassak, 1993).

Surveys comparing conventional low back care with chiropractic care show equally dramatic results. In a 1989 survey of members of an health maintenance organization in Washington that offers both conventional and chiropractic care, 359 low back patients of conventional doctors were compared to 348 patients who used chiropractic. Chiropractic patients were three times as likely as patients of family physicians to report that they were very satisfied with the care they received for low back pain (66% versus 22%) (Cherkin and MacCornack, 1989). The only other such comparative study, done in Utah in 1973 in patients with low back pain, had a similiar outcome in terms of satisfaction (Kane *et al.*, 1974). Self-selected patients who were interviewed retrospectively are getting something from chiropractic in a magnitude seemingly higher than the Meade study (1990).

Bayesian efficacy: an emerging perspective

One approach to efficacy that has been lacking in the complementary and alternative medicine literature and has only begun to have a serious impact on conventional discussion is the Bayesian approach. Deriving from the early statistical work of Thomas Bayes (1701–1761), this alternative approach to efficacy attempts to blend the strengths of the other three approaches and offset the limitations. This approach incorporates prior beliefs expressed as probabilities and clinical information into the question of evaluating results from studies. The Bayesian analytical approach has formed the basis of clinical decision analysis for the past two decades (Weinstein and Fineberg, 1980) and is recently being applied to the analysis of clinical trials (Browner and Newman, 1987; Hughs, 1993; Lewis and Wears, 1993; Brophy and Joseph, 1995). Brophy and Joseph (1995) applied a Bayesian approach to the GUSTO study of various thrombolytic strategies in acute myocardial infarction and concluded that: 'Standard statistical analyses of randomized clinical trials fail to provide a direct assessment of which treatment is superior or the probability of a clinically meaningful difference. A Bayesian analysis permits the calculation of the probability that a treatment is superior based on the observed data and prior beliefs. The subjectivity of prior beliefs in the Bayesian approach is not a liability, but rather explicitly allows different opinions to be formally expressed and evaluated' (Brophy and Joseph, 1995).

This alternative way of analysing and interpreting clinical trial results has been available for a number of years but has not been widely adopted because it is based on a different set of assumptions to classical statistical analyses and trials. Knowledge and beliefs regarding effectiveness prior to the trial *and* the trial data results both matter rather than the classical assumption of a null hypothesis of no difference. Browner and Newman (1987) make the analogy between diagnostic tests and research studies in stating that, 'the interpretation of a test result depends on characteristics of both the test and the patient being tested ... knowing the specificity and sensitivity of a diagnostic test is necessary, but insufficient; the clinician must also estimate the prior probability of the disease'. The Bayesian assumptions are consistent with everyday clinical practice. 'The Bayesian approach is more consistent with clinicians' common sense method of reasoning and emphasizes the estimation of effect magnitude rather than the artificiality of hypothesis testing' (Lewis and Wears, 1993). In this regard, the Bayesian approach resembles pragmatic efficacy in its emphasis on clinical relevance. It also attempts to incorporate the prior belief component that is the keystone of the performative approach. The Bayesian approach also leaves room for the methods of a fastidious approach but the uses of the outcome of those methods are tempered by incorporating the pragmatic and performative aspects. A complete comparison of Bayesian versus classical approaches is in Lewis and Wears (1993), Brophy and Joseph (1995), Hughs (1993) and beyond the scope of this chapter. We are introducing this approach because a serious consideration may be helpful to a review of complementary and alternative medicine efficacy in future work.

In addition to the cultural barriers associated with adopting a new approach, there are several limitations to the Bayesian approach. The first relates to the quantification of prior beliefs. Quantification is expensive, subject to biases, and requires constant updating (Slovic, Fischhoff and Lichtenstein, 1980; Kahneman, Slovic and Tversky, 1982). However, since prior beliefs exist anyway, the decision becomes a matter of how we include them – not if they exist. The response to the homoeopathy trials is evidence of the role of prior beliefs that need to be explicitly included in the research and interpretation of the research process. A second limitation is that Bayesian analysis is often computationally complex; however, the greatly expanded powers of computers ease this burden. The third limitation is that a Bayesian approach shifts more responsibility to the readers and users of the trial results; however, they may not want this responsibility. Some readers and users may resist the additional effort required by a Bayesian approach; but the extra effort makes the biases explicit rather than implicit on the experimenters' part.

Implications of a Bayesian approach for efficacy beyond placebo

The Bayesian approach has implications for answering this question on four levels: the individual patient level; the interpretation of studies and use of study results level; the pooling of study results level; and how one asks and answers the question of efficacy beyond placebo level.

At the patient level, a patient's prior beliefs affect his or her health outcome and patient-provider dynamics affect the patient's outcome. However, studies do not control for these aspects and, therefore, the results are essentially random or uninterpretable because providers and provider-patient pairings are not randomized. Furthermore, the act of randomization might actually change the outcome because of the unclear impact of randomization on a particular patient's beliefs.

In terms of the interpretation of studies, evidence already shows that the effects of research studies on clinical practice are wide. Boissel (1989) concluded that, '. . . studies on the impact of RCTs (randomized clinical trials) on medical practice have shown large and frequent discrepancies between scientific data made available from RCTs and current prescription practices in France, the United States, Finland, Holland, and elsewhere'. Each user of the research results is implicitly applying his or her prior beliefs to any research results that he or she might come in contact with. The Bayesian approach allows this implicit action to become explicit.

The pooling of studies and the biases of those doing the pooling further compound the problems noted at the individual patient level and the interpretation of a single study level. The Limberg group's meta-analysis of homoeopathy demonstrated how prior beliefs implicitly affect 'objective' reviews and meta-analysis. Since no one can escape his or her prior beliefs, it becomes impossible to be purely 'objective'; therefore, it becomes imperative to make those beliefs explicit to foster the highest quality of scientific communication possible.

Finally, to answer the question of efficacy beyond placebo, a Bayesian would ask what are the prior beliefs regarding efficacy beyond placebo. If one believes non-specific effects are an inseparable concept in practice (only separable in theory and discussion at best), then the question is rendered irrelevant. If one believes non-specific effects can be separated, then the ethics and implementation in a specific clinical trial drive the answer. For example, therapy A works (does not work) beyond placebo in x condition for y type of patients under z circumstances. Since the answer is a blend of prior beliefs and study results, then the effect of one's prior belief is larger when trial results are weak and unconvincing (Lewis and Wears, 1993). Since the evidence for efficacy beyond placebo is equivocal for many complementary and alternative medicine therapies, then one's prior belief regarding the answer becomes the answer at this stage of the research.

Conclusion

The question of whether or not complementary and alternative medicine has efficacy beyond the placebo has been approached from three perspectives. In the fastidious model, it seems that a definitive answer has not been provided for many people (even when there is some good evidence, as in the case of homoeopathy). Many methodological problems need to be clarified before this method will produce definitive answers.

The pragmatic model circumvents the question of efficacy beyond placebo and has provided evidence that there is a significant total outcome effect for chiropractic and manual therapy concerning low back pain. Whether this effect is a verum-specific effect, a mega-placebo effect, or a combination of verum-specific and non-specific effects cannot be answered within this model.

The performative model demonstrates that for scientifically naive, ordinary people complementary and alternative medicine has an obvious and clearly demonstrable value. It is likely that if these people were asked 'is there efficacy beyond placebo?' that they would respond from their own clear experience that complementary and alternative medicine has efficacy beyond the sham (placebo).

Finally, the Bayesian model provides one option for integrating some aspects of all three approaches to answering the question of efficacy beyond placebo.

References

Anderson, D. C., Jamieson, J. L. and Man, S. C. (1974) Analgesic effects of acupuncture on the pain of ice water: a double-blind study. *Canadian Journal of Psychology*, **28**, 239–244

Anthony, H. M. (1993) Some methodological problems in the assessment of complementary therapy. In: *Clinical Research Methodology For Complementary Therapies*, edited by G. T. Lewith and D. Aldridge. London: Hodder & Stoughton

Assendelft, W. J. J., Koes, B. W., van de Heijden, G. J. M. G. and Bouter, L. M. (1992) The efficacy of chiropractic manipulation of back pain: blinded review of relevant randomized clinical trials. *Journal of Manipulation and Physiological Therapeutics*, **15**, 487–494

Barry, M. J., Fowler, F. J., Mulley, A. G. Jr, Henderson, J. V. Jr and Wennberg, J. E. (1995) Patient reactions to a program designed to facilitate participation in treatment decisions for benign prostatic hyperplasia. *Medical Care*, **33**, 771–782

Beecher, H. K. (1955) The powerful placebo. *Journal of the American Medical Association*, **159**, 1602–1606

Bergmann, J. F. (1994) A randomised clinical trial of the effect of informed consent on the analgesic activity of placebo and naproxen in cancer pain. *Clinical Trials and Meta-Analysis*, **29**, 41–47

Bergquist-Ullman, M. and Larsson, U. (1977) Acute low back pain in industry. *Acta Orthopaedica Scandinavica* Supp 10, 1–117

Bigos, S. J., Bowyer, O. R., Braen, G. R., Brown, K., Deyo, R., Halfeman, S. *et al.* (1994) *Clinical Practice Guideline. Number 14. Acute Low Back Problems in Adults.* Rockville, MD: Agency for Health Care Policy and Research, US DHHS

Boissel, J. P. (1989) Impact of randomized clinical trials on medical practices. *Controlled Clinical Trials*, **10**, 120S–134S

British Homoeopathic Journal (1943) Editorial. The mustard gas experiments. **23**, 131–142

Brophy, J. M. and Joseph, L. (1995) Placing trials in context using bayesian analysis. *Journal of the American Medical Association*, **273**, 871–875

Browner, W. S. and Newman, T. B. (1987) Are all significant p values created equal?

The analogy between diagnostic tests and clinical research. *Journal of the American Medical Association*, **257**, 2459–2463

Cassedy, J. H. (1984) *American Medicine and Statistical Thinking, 1800–1860*. Cambridge, Massachusetts: Harvard University Press

Cherkin, D. C. and MacCornack, F. A. (1989) Patient evaluation of low back pain care from family physicians and chiropractors. *Western Journal of Medicine*, **150**, 351–355

Csordas, T. J. (1983) The rhetoric of transformation in ritual healing. *Culture, Medicine and Psychiatry*, **7**, 333–375

Csordas, T. J. (1994) *The Sacred Self: A Cultural Phenomenology of Charismatic Healing*. Berkeley: University of California Press

Dahan, R. (1986) Does informed consent influence therapeutic outcome? A clinical trial of the hypnotic activity of placebo in patients admitted to hospital. *British Medical Journal*, **293**, 363–364

Dimond, E. G., Kittle, F. and Crockett, J. E. (1960) Comparison of internal mammary artery ligation and sham operation for angina pectoris. *American Journal of Cardiology*, 383–386

Eisenberg, D. (1995) Traditional Chinese Medicine. In: *Alternative Medicine: Implications for Clinical Practice*. Boston: Harvard Medical School, Dept. of Continuing Education

Eisenberg, D., Kessler, R. C., Foster, C., Norlock, F. G., Culkins, D. R., Delbenco, T. L. (1993) Unconventional medicine in the United States. Prevalence, costs, and pattern use. *New England Journal of Medicine*, **328**, 246–252

Ernst, E. (1995) Patient's perception of complementary therapies. Forsch. *Komplementärmed.*, **2**: 326–29.

Evan, W. and Hoyle, C. (1933) The comparative value of drugs used in the continuous treatment of angina pectoris. *Quarterly Journal of Medicine*, **26**, 311–338.

Feinstein, A. R. (1985) *Clinical Epidemiology*. Philadephia: W. B. Saunders

Gibson, T., Harkness, J., Blagrave, P., Grahame, G., Woo, P., Hills, P. (1984) Controlled comparison of short-wave diathermy treatment with osteopathic treatment in non-specific low back pain. *Lancet*, **i(8440)**, 1258–1261

Glover, J. R., Morris, J. G. and Kholsa, T. (1974) Back pain: a randomized clinical trial of rotational manipulation of the trunk. *British Journal of Industrial Medicine*, **31**, 59–64

Godfrey, C. M., Morgan, P. P. and Schatzker, J. (1984) A randomized trial of manipulation for low-back pain in a medical setting. *Spine*, **9**, 301–304

Gold, H., Kwit, N. T. and Otto, H. (1937) The xanthines (theobromine and aminophylline) in the treatment of cardiac pain. *Journal of the American Medical Association*, **108**, 2173–2179

Gotzsche, P. C. (1994) Is there logic in the placebo? *Lancet*, **ii**, 925–926

Gracely, R. H., Dubner, R., Decter, W. R. and Wolskee, P. J. (1985) Clinician's expectations influence placebo analgesia (Letter). *Lancet*, **i**, 43

Greenfield, S. (1989) The state of outcomes research: are we on target? *New England Journal of Medicine*, **320**, 1142–1143

Harris, L. and Associates (1987) *Health, Information and the Use of Questionable Treatments: A Study of the American Public*. Washington, DC: US Dept. of Health and Human Services

Hill, C. and Doyon, F. (1990) Review of randomized trials of homoeopathy. *Revue D'Epidemilogie et de Sante Publique*, **38**, 139–147

Henshaw, R. C., Naji, S. A., Russell, I. T., Templeton, A. A. (1993) Comparison of medical abortion with surgical vacuum aspiration: women's preferences and acceptability of treatment. *British Medical Journal*, **307**, 714–717

Hoehler, F. K., Tobis, J. S. and Buerger, A. A. (1981) Spinal manipulation of low back pain. *Journal of the American Medical Association*, **245**, 1835–1838

Hogben, L. and Sim, M. (1953) The self-controlled and self-recorded clinical trial for low-grade morbidity. *British Journal of Preventive Social Medicine*, **7**, 163–179

Hughs, M. D. (1993) Reporting bayesian analysis of clinical trials. *Statistics in Medicine*, **12**, 1651–1663

Hughes, J. R., Gulliver, S. B., Amori, G. *et al.* (1989) Effect of instruction and nicotine on smoking cessation withdrawal symptoms and self-administration of nicotine gum. *Psychopharmacology*, **99**, 486–491

Hull, J. G. and Bond, C. F. (1986) Social and behavioral consequences of alcohol consumption and expectancy: a meta-analysis. *Psychological Bulletin*, **99**, 347–360

Idler, E. L. and Kasl, S. (1991) Health perceptions and survival: do global evaluations of health status really predict mortality? *Journal of Gerontology*, **46**, S55–65

Jensen, M. P. and Karoly, P. (1991) Motivation and expectancy factor in symptom perception: a laboratory study of the placebo effect. *Psychosomatic Medicine*, **53**, 144–152

Kahneman, D., Slovic, P. and Tversky, A. (1982) *Judgement under Uncertainty: Heuristics and Biases*. Cambridge: Cambridge University Press

Kane, R. L., Leymaster, C., Olsow, D. and Woolley, F. R. (1974) Manipulating the patient: a comparison of the effectiveness of physician and chiropractic care. *Lancet*, **i**, 1333–1336

Kaufman, M. (1971) *Homeopathy in America: The Rise and Fall of a Medical Heresy*. Baltimore: The Johns Hopkins University Press

King, L. S. (1991) *Transformations in American Medicine*. Baltimore: The Johns Hopkins University Press

Kirmayer, L. J. (1993) Healing and the invention of metaphor: the effectiveness of symbols revisited. *Culture, Medicine and Psychiatry*, **17**, 161–195

Kirsch, I. and Rosadino, M. J. (1993) Do double-blind studies with informed consent yield externally valid results? *Psychopharmacology*, **110**, 437–442

Kirsch, I. and Weixel, L. J. (1988) Double-blind versus deceptive administration of a placebo. *Behavioral Neuroscience*, **102**, 319–323

Kleijnen, J., Knipschild, P. and ter Riet, G. (1991) Clinical trials of homeopathy. *British Medical Journal*, **302**, 316–323

Kleijnen, J, de Craen, A. J. M., van Everdingen, J. and Krol, L. (1994) Placebo effect in double-blind clinical trials: a review of interactions with medications. *Lancet*, **ii**, 1347–1349

Klienman, A. (1973) Medicine's symbolic reality: on a central problem in the philosophy of medicine. *Inquiry*, **16**, 206–213

Koes, B. W., Bouter, L. M., vanMameren, H., Essers, A. H. M., Verstegen, G. J. M. G., Hofhuizen, D. M., *et al.* (1992) Randomized clinical trial of manipulative therapy and physiotherapy for persistent back and neck complaints: results of one year follow up. *British Medical Journal*, **304**, 601–605

Koes, B. W., Bouter, L. M. and vanMameren, H., Essers, A. H. M., Verstegen, G. J. M. G., Hofhuizen, D. M. *et al.* (1993) A randomized clinical trial of manual therapy and physiotherapy for persistent back and neck complaints: subgroup analysis and relationship between outcome measures. *Journal of Manipulative and Physiological Therapeutics*, **16**, 211–219

Ledermann, E. K. (1954) Homoeopathy tested against controls in cases of surgical tuberculosis. *British Homoeopathic Journal*, **44**, 83–96

Lewis, R. J. and Wears, R. L. (1993) An introduction to the bayesian analysis of clinical trials. *Annals of Emergency Medicine*, **22**, 1328–1336

Lewith, G. T. and Machin, M. (1983) On the evaluation of clinical effects of acupuncture. *Pain*, **16**, 111–127

Lilienfeld, A. M. (1982) Ceteris paribus: the evolution of the clinical trial. *Bulletin of Historical Medicine*, **56**, 1–18

Llewellyn-Thomas, H. A. (1991) Patients' willingness to enter clinical trials: measuring the association with perceived benefit and preference for decision participation. *Social Science and Medicine*, **32**, 35–42

Louis, T. A. and Shapiro, S. H. (1983) Critical issues in the conduct and interpretation of clinical trials. *Annual Review of Public Health*, **4**, 25–46

Lyon, M. L. (1990) Order and healing: the concept of order and its importance in the conceptualization of healing. *Medical Anthropology*, **12**, 249–268

McConnell, J. D., Barry, M. J., Bruskewitz, R. C., Bueschev, A. J., Denton, S. E., Holtgrewe, H. L. *et al.* (1994) *Clinical Practice Guidelines. Number 8. Benign Prostatic Hyperplasia: Diagnosis and Treatment.* Rockville, MD: Agency for Health Care Policy and Research, US DHHS

Man, S. C. and Baragar, F. D. (1974) Preliminary clinical study of acupuncture in rheumatoid arthritis. *Journal of Rheumatology*, **1**, 126–129

Meade, T. W., Dyer, S., Browne, W., Townsend, J. and Frank, A. D. (1990) Low back pain of mechanical origin: randomised comparison of chiropractic and hospital outpatient treatment. *British Medical Journal*, **300**, 1431–1437

Meade, T. W., Dyer, S., Browne, W. and Frank, A. O. (1995) Randomized comparison of chiropractic and hospital outpatient management for low back pain: results from extended follow-up. *British Journal of Medicine*, **311**, 349–51

Myers, M. G., Cairns, J. A. and Singer, J. (1987) The consent form as a possible cause of side effects. *Clinical Pharmacology and Therapeutics*, **42**, 250–253

Morgan, J. P., Dickey, J. L., Hunt, H. H. and Hudgins, P. M. (1985) A controlled trial of spinal manipulation in the management of hypertension. *Journal of the American Osteopathy Association*, **85**, 308–313

Ongley M. J., Klien, R. G., Dorman, T. A., Eek, B. C., Hubert, L. J. (1987) A new approach to the treatment of chronic low back pain. *Lancet*, **ii**, 143–146

Oths, K. (1994) Communication in a chiropractic clinic: how a DC treats his patient. *Culture Medicine and Psychiatry*, **18**, 83–113

Ottenbacher, K. (1992) Impact of random assignment on study outcome: an empirical examination. *Controlled Clinical Trials*, **13**, 50–61

Patel M., Gutzwiller, F., Paccaud, F., Marazzi, A. (1989) A meta-analysis of acupuncture for chronic pain. *International Journal of Epidemiology*, **18**, 900–904

Paterson, J. (1944) Report on mustard gas experiments. *Journal of the American Institute of Homeopathy*, **37**, 47–50

Penick, S. B. and Fisher, S. (1965) Drug-set interaction: psychological and physiological effects of epinephrine under differential expectations. *Psychosomatic Medicine*, **27**, 177–182

Penick, S. and Hinkle, L. (1964) The effect of expectation on response to phenmetrazine. *Psychosomatic Medicine*, **24**, 369–73

Pocock, S. J. (1985) Current issues in the design and interpretation of clinical trials. *British Medical Journal*, **290**, 39–42

Reilly, R. P. and Findley, T. W. (1989) Research in physical medicine and rehabilitation. *American Journal of Physiological Medicine and Rehabilitation*, **68**, 196–201

Rogers, W. J. (1994) What is the optimal tool to define appropriate therapy: the randomized clinical trial, meta-analysis, or outcomes research? *Current Opinion in Cardiology*, **9**, 401–403

Rosner, B. (1995) *Fundamentals of Biostatistics*, 4th edn. Belmont, MA: Duxbury Press

Sarles, E., Camatte, R. and Sahel, J. (1977) A study of the variations in the response regarding duodenal ulcer when treated by placebo by different investigators. *Digestion*, **16**, 289–292

Sawyer, C. E. and Kassak, K. (1993) Patient satisfaction with chiropractic care. *Journal of Manipulative and Physiological Therapeutics*, **16**, 25–32

Schwartz, D. and Lellouch, J. (1967) Explanatory and pragmatic attitudes in therapeutical trials. *Journal of Chronic Diseases*, **20**, **8**, 637–648

Shekelle, P. G., Adams, A. H., Chessin, M. R., Hurwitz, E. L. and Brook, R. H. (1992) Spinal manipulation for low-back pain. *Annals of Internal Medicine*, **117**, 590–598

Skovlund, E. (1991) Should we tell trial patients that they might receive placebo? (Letter). *Lancet*, **i**, 1041

Sims-Williams, H., Jayson, M. I. V., Young, S. M., Buddeley, H. and Collins, E. (1978) Controlled trial of mobilization and manipulation for patients with low back pain in general practice. *British Medical Journal*, **2**, 1338–1340

Sims-Williams *et al.* (1979) Controlled trial of mobilization and manipulation for low back pain: hospital patients. *British Medical Journal*, **2**, 1318–1320

Slovic, P., Fischhoff, B. and Lichtenstein, S. (1980) Facts and fears: understanding perceived risk. In: *Societal Risk Assessment: How Safe is Safe Enough?* edited by R. C. Schwing and W. A. Albers Jr. New York: Plenum Press

Sox, H. C., Margulies, I. and Sox, C. H. (1981) Psychologically mediated effects of diagnostic tests. *Annals of Internal Medicine*, **95**, 680–685

Spilker, B. (1991) *Guide to Clinical Trials*. New York: Raven Press

Sullivan, M. D. (1993) Placebo controls and epistemic control in orthodox medicine. *Journal of Medical Philosophy*, **18**, 213–231

Tambiah, S. J. (1990) *Magic, Science, Religion, and the Scope of Rationality.* Cambridge: Cambridge University Press

Tauber, A. I. (1994) Darwinian aftershocks: repercussions in late twentieth century medicine. *Journal of the Royal Society of Medicine*, **87**, 27–31

ter Riet, G., Kleijnen, J. and Knipschild, P. (1990) Acupuncture and chronic pain: a criteria-based meta-analysis. *Journal of Clinical Epidemiology*, **43**, 1191–1199

Turner, J. L., Gallimore, R. and Fox-Henning, C. (1980) An annotated bibliography of placebo research. *Journal of Supplementary Abstracts of the American Psychology Association*, **10**, 1–296

Uhlenhuth, E. H., Richels, K., Fisher, S., Park, L. C., Lipman, R. S., Mock, J. (1966) Drug, doctor's verbal attitude and clinic seting in the symptomatic response to pharmacotherapy. *Psychopharmacologia*, **9**, 392–418

Vickers, A. (1995) External validity in homoeopathic research. *British Homoeopathic Journal*, **85**, 95–101

Waagen, G. N., Haldeman, S., Cook, G., Lopez, D., De Boer, K. F. (1986) Short term trial of chiropractic adjustments for the relief of chronic low back pain. *Manual Medicine*, **2**, 63–67

Vincent, C. and Lewith, G. (1995) Placebo controls for acupuncture studies. *Journal of the Royal Society of Medicine*, **88**, 199–202

Wardwell, W. I. (1989) The Connecticut survey of public attitudes toward chiropractic. *Journal of Manipulative and Physiological Therapeutics*, **12**, 109–21

Weinstein, M. C. and Fineberg, H. V. (1980) *Clinical Decision Analysis*. Philadelphia: W. B. Saunders

Wennberg, J. E. (1990) What is outcomes research? In: *Modern Methods of Clinical Investigation*, edited by A. C. Gelijns. Washington, D.C: National Academy Press

White, L., Tursky, B. and Schwartz, G. E. (1985) *Placebo: Theory, Research and Mechanisms*. New York: Guilford Press

Williamson, J. W., Goldschmidt, P. G. and Colton, T. (1986) The quality of medical literature: an analysis of validation assessments. In: *Medical Uses of Statistics*, edited by J. C. Bailer and F. Mosteller. Waltham, MA: NEJM Books. pp. 370–391

Wolf, S. (1950) Effects of suggestion and conditioning on the action of chemical agents in human subjects – the pharmacology of placebos. *Journal of Clinical Investigation*, **29**, 100–109

Wolf, S. (1962) Part IV. Placebos: problems and pitfalls. *Clinical Pharmacology and Therapeutics*, **3**, 254–257

Yates, R. L., Lamping, D. L., Abram, N. L. and Wright, C. (1988) Effects of chiropractic treatment on blood pressure and anxiety: a randomized, controlled trial. *Journal of Manipulative and Physiological Therapeutics*, **11**, 484–488.

Chapter 5

Why do people choose and use complementary therapies?

Adrian Furnham

Introduction

The question, which is the title of this chapter, may, to some, seem impertinent. Have people, it may be asked, ever posed the question why choose and use orthodox medicine? The lay person would, no doubt, believe this a pointless question with a self-evident answer. One consults (chooses and uses) an orthodox medical expert for advice and help (diagnosis and cure). The fact that one might pose the question why use complementary therapies must therefore imply that they may be used for other reasons, or indeed that the act of choosing a complementary practitioner is not altogether wise or safe.

This chapter reviews the growing, but as yet fairly limited, literature on how orthodox and complementary patients differ in an attempt to understand why they chose one over the other. Various hypo-theses have been proposed for why some people are attracted to or shun the increasingly diverse range of complementary medicines (Bakx, 1991; Baum, 1989; Bowling, 1994; Calnan, 1987; Cart and Calnan, 1991).

According to Helman (1990), some individuals tend to act as a source of health advice more often than others. These include those with a long experience of particular illness, or type of treatment; those with extensive experience of certain life events, such as women who have raised several children; the paramedical professions (such as nurses, pharmacists, physiotherapists or doctor's receptionists) who are consulted informally about health problems; doctors' wives or husbands, who share some of their spouses' experience, if not training; individuals such as chiropodists, hairdressers, or even bank managers who interact frequently with the public and sometimes act as lay confessors or psychotherapists; the organizers of self-help groups; and the members or officials of certain healing cults or churches. These advisors' credentials are mainly their own experience rather than education, social status or special expertise. This list omits the complementary medicine practitioners, both those from the more established, and those from the newer areas of therapy.

Many forms of complementary (alternative) medicine have long histories. Herbs have been used medicinally for at least 5000 years and acupuncture for at least 2000 years. Homoeopathy derives from the work of Samuel Hahnemann, who published his *Materia Medica* in 1811. Osteopathy also developed in the nineteenth century. Given the achievements of modern orthodox medicine, one might have expected that these earlier forms of medicine would have passed into obscurity. However, in the last 25 years, interest in complementary medicine has increased steadily and has been especially rapid over the last decade (Research Council for Complementary Medicine, 1994). This growth of interest has also led to more research into the efficacy of complementary medicine and changing attitudes towards it (Fitzpatrick, 1984; Fulder and Munro, 1985; Wharton and Lewith, 1986; Furnham and Smith, 1988; Vincent, Furnham and Willsmore, 1995; Sharma, 1992).

Complementary (alternative) medicine is now widely used throughout the developed world. The major complementary therapies, such as acupuncture, homoeopathy, herbalism and osteopathy, are extensively used and increasingly accepted (BMA, 1993). In the UK, Fulder and Munro (1985) found that in 1981 complementary consultations averaged 19 500 per 100 000 people – 6.5% of general practice consultations. Acupuncture, chiropractic and osteopathy were the most popular specialities with about two million consultations each year. Overall about 1.5 million people (2.5% of the population) were receiving courses of treatment in a single year. This has probably grown in the intervening period. Thomas *et al.* (1987) estimated that their more restricted group of professionally registered complementary practitioners undertook four million consultations per year, roughly one for every 55 patient consultations with an NHS general practitioner.

In Europe, studies suggest that between one-third and one-half of the adult population have used complementary medicine at some time. Where self-medication with homoeopathic and herbal remedies is included in the definition (for studies in Belgium, Finland and France), approximately one-third of people have had some complementary treatment in the previous year (Lewith and Aldridge, 1991; Sharma, 1992). In the USA, Eisenberg, Kessler and Foster (1993) have recently found that more visits are made to providers of 'unconventional' therapy (which includes the more widely known complementary therapies) than to all USA primary care physicians (general practitioners). The expenditure on unconventional therapies was comparable to that spent on all hospitalizations in the USA. Eisenberg's definition ('commonly used interventions neither taught widely in USA medical schools nor generally available in USA hospitals') included all the major complementary therapies, vitamin and mineral supplements, and other complementary remedies. Also included however were taking exercise and relaxation techniques – hardly unconventional therapies. The results exaggerate the use of truly unconventional therapies, but nevertheless show a widespread use and acceptance. Thus although all data in this area are both unreliable and confounded, it appears that rather than see the slow demise of complementary medicine in the face of advancements in orthodox clinical medicine, the opposite appears to be the case.

The reasons for this increased interest and use of complementary medicine are not well understood, though many opinions have been offered. Some have suggested that the move towards complementary medicine represents a 'flight from science' (Smith, 1983) or credulous faith in occult or paranormal phenomena (Skrabanek, 1988; Baum, 1989). In one small empirical study, a survey of 65 patients attending a clinic of complementary medicine found that the failure of conventional medicine (for their complaint) was the main reason for attending (Moore et al., 1985). In all studies, patients using complementary or unconventional therapies tend to be those with relatively more education and higher incomes (Sharma, 1992). These results are 'not compatible with a picture of a patient unable to understand the medical possibilities or to make discriminating choices' (Fulder and Munro, 1985). Furthermore, it is becoming clear that it is relatively rare for complementary patients to abandon orthodox medicine. Complementary therapies, which are generally used for chronic, as opposed to life-threatening, conditions are generally used as an adjunct to conventional treatment, rather than as a replacement for it (Thomas et al., 1991). Patients seem rather to consider a range of therapeutic options including self-medication, complementary medicine and conventional treatment and will make use of different forms of medicine on different occasions (Thomas et al., 1991; Eisenberg, Kessler and Foster, 1993). The average patient has a discriminating mix and match, rather than an either/or approach to seeking advice and treatment for their ailments.

There are a number of possible reasons for turning to complementary medicine. Some patients are 'pushed' because they may have become dissatisfied with orthodox medicine, rejecting its reliance on high technology and wary of the dangers of invasive techniques and the toxicity of many drugs. Others are 'pulled' because while they may retain a belief in the value and effectiveness of orthodox medicine, at least in certain areas, they may find some aspects of complementary medicine attractive. They may regard it as especially efficacious for some conditions, and dealing more with the emotional aspects of the illness, or as having a spiritual dimension that is not seen as important in orthodox medicine.

Suffice it to say that there is no prototype complementary medicine patient. It is probably rare to find patients that always choose to be exclusive to a type, or a number of different types, of complementary medicine. Most patients 'shop' for treatment. Cultural, educational and ideological factors affect choice, but also access and availability, as well, of course, as the acute and chronic nature of their illness. That is, in some countries, certain types of therapies abound, while in others they are comparatively rare and not highly thought of.

Programmatic studies

Over the past decade, a series of programmatic studies has been performed that has examined how patients of orthodox medicine and the most established complementary medicine specialities differ. In a way, they have all attempted to answer the question 'why do patients choose to visit particular specialists?'. Furnham and Smith (1988) compared two groups of patients, one visiting a general practitioner and the other a homoeopath, who were not significantly different in terms of sex, age, education, marital status, religion and income. They were asked to complete a questionnaire, measuring such things as their perceived susceptibility to disease and illness; their beliefs concerning their self-control over health; measures of their own mental health; preventative measures in staying healthy and the perceived efficacy of orthodox versus complementary treatment. The major differences between the two groups were the fact that the homoeopathic group were much more critical and sceptical about the efficacy of orthodox medicine; they believed that their general health could be improved; and they tended to have higher psychiatric morbidity. By and large, the two groups did not differ in their beliefs about illness susceptibility or preventative measures.

Furnham and Bhagrath (1992) continued this research with a second, related study. Two samples of patients were chosen, one from a general practitioner's surgery and the other from an outpatient department at a homoeopathic hospital. Both groups were then asked to fill out a questionnaire measuring health consciousness, risk and prevention, health beliefs, medical history and mental health. It was found that the homoeopathic sample were far more dissatisfied with orthodox medicine than the general practitioner sample, and this, rather than a strong belief in the complementary therapy, was their major reason for visiting a homoeopath. It was also found that they were more aware of preventative health measures and had an increased incidence of psychiatric morbidity. The two groups did not differ in their beliefs of getting, and susceptibility to, diseases.

The results suggested that the homoeopathic group were more aware and conscious of their health, and had a greater belief in the underlying exposition of homoeopathy, and that they chose homoeopathy because of some experience of unsatisfactory orthodox medical care.

Furnham and Forey (1994) were also concerned with different health and illness beliefs of patients choosing orthodox versus complementary medicine. Two groups of patients, one visiting a general practitioner and the other a homoeopath, were not significantly different in terms of age, sex, level of education, marital status, occupational status, political views, newspaper readership, ethnic grouping, how religious they were and income. They were asked to complete a fairly long and extensive questionnaire measuring such factors as their beliefs concerning control over their health; preventative and restorative measures in staying healthy; perceived efficacy of orthodox versus complementary medicine treatment; type of therapies they have tried; types of illness they believe benefit from either of both types of practice; and physiological location and function. Results showed that the complementary medicine group were more critical and sceptical about the efficacy of orthodox medicine; they believed more than the general practitioner group that their health could be improved; they stayed more loyal to their chosen practitioner; they had tried more complementary therapies and had more self- and ecologically aware lifestyles than the general practitioner group; they believed that treatment should concentrate on the whole person and possessed greater knowledge of the physiology of the body than the patients of orthodox medicine. The results suggested that people who choose complementary medicine may do so not from disenchantment with, and bad experience of, orthodox medical practitioners, but rather from a belief in the effectiveness of complementary medicine and principles and practices.

Furnham and Kirkcaldy (1996) replicated the study in Germany. The study examined different attitudes towards health and illness among an adult, working, German population. Two hundred and two subjects completed a questionnaire which assessed such beliefs as control over one's health; preventative and restorative measures in staying healthy; perceived efficacy of orthodox versus complementary medicine treatment; the underlying physiological or psychological bases of illnesses, and health consciousness. There was some evidence that women were more inclined to attend complementary forms of treatment, and that younger persons were more likely to consult an orthodox general practitioner, otherwise demographic variables were unrelated to preference for orthodox or complementary forms of treatment. Overall, the complementary medicine group compared with the general practitioner group were more critical and sceptical of the effectiveness of orthodox medicine; they felt their health could be improved; they were more loyal to their practitioner; and appeared to display more ecologically aware lifestyles. Again these results indicated clients who select complementary forms of treatment may do so less from disenchantment with, and bad experience of, orthodox medical techniques, but rather from a deep seated belief in the effectiveness of complementary medicine.

In a recent British study that examined the beliefs and behaviours of three groups of complementary medicine and a general practice group of patients, Furnham, Vincent and Wood (1995) asked patients ($n = 256$) consulting either a general practitioner or one of three complementary practitioners, (osteopath, homoeopath or acupuncturist) to complete a seven-part questionnaire which looked at demographic data, medical history, familiarization with complementary therapies, health beliefs and lifestyles, health locus of control, scientific health beliefs and their perceptions of the consultation style of general and complementary practitioners. The four subject groups did not differ significantly in the demographic variables of sex, years of schooling, whether or not they had a degree, marital status, or income, but did differ on age and number of children. The effects of both the significant demographic variables and some aspects of patients' medical history were controlled for subsequent analyses because they could have accounted for any differences found between the four groups' beliefs and behaviours. Acupuncture patients stood out as having the most different chronic medical history compared to the other three groups who were fairly similar to each other. They were also least satisfied with their general practitioners, had least confidence in prescribed drugs and were most concerned with leading a healthy lifestyle. The acupuncture patients were most sceptical about orthodox medicine. The main finding was that patients of complementary practitioners are not a homogeneous group but do differ in their views on satisfaction with general practitioners, healthy lifestyle, global environmental issues, confidence in prescribed drugs, faith in medical science, importance of a 'healthy mind', harmful effects of medical science, and scientific methodology. The results imply that patients consult different practitioners, general or alternative, on the basis of a combination of their level of scepticism about orthodox medicine, their lifestyle and other health beliefs.

Vincent and Furnham (1996) asked over 250 patients from three complementary medical practices (acupuncture, osteopathy and homoeopathy) why they chose their particular practitioner (Table 5.1). Of the twenty reasons they were presented with, the patients agreed strongly with almost one-third. The reasons that were most strongly endorsed were 'because I value the emphasis on treating the whole person'; 'because I believe complementary therapy will be more effective for my problem than orthodox medicine'; 'because I believe that complementary medicine will enable me to take a more active part in maintaining my health' and 'because orthodox treatment was not effective for my particular problem'. There was little difference between the groups on their rating of the most important reasons.

The least important reasons rated by the groups included 'because complementary treatment is less expensive than orthodox private medicine' and 'because I value a form of therapy that actually involves touching me'. Curiously, there were significant differences between the groups on these reasons; the acupuncturists rated costs as much less important than did the homoeopathic patients, in spite of the fact that the homoeopathy patients were attending a National Health Service Hospital. The homoeopathy group rated the fact that their chosen therapy allowed them a more active part in their health more highly than the osteopathy group, suggesting that a discussion of diet and lifestyle factors may play a stronger role in homoeopathic consultations. Patients did not perceive orthodox medicine as generally ineffective, indicating that they are not suffering from a wholesale disillusion with medicine. Orthodox medicine is only seen as ineffective for their specific problem.

The factor analysis of the twenty reasons gave fairly clear results which underpinned many speculations from researchers in this field (Table 5.2). The first, most important, factor was clearly a 'pull' factor which included items that stressed that complementary treatment was more natural, effective, relaxing, sensible and that one could take an active part in it. The second, with almost equal importance, was the specific failure of orthodox medicine to bring them relief. The third factor was also a specific 'push' factor which primarily concerned poor communication between patients and orthodox medicine practitioners. The fourth was a highly specific 'push' factor which primarily concerned poor communication between patients and orthodox medicine practitioners. The fifth, relatively unimportant factor stressed the easy, cost-effective and available nature of complementary therapies. Clearly these different factors, although not strongly distinguished between the three complementary therapies, are likely to differ in importance for each individual according to their specific medical history, personal beliefs and temperament.

Three of the factors showed significant differences between the three patient groups. Acupuncture and homoeopathy patients seemed put off by the potential side effects of medicine more than the osteopathy group. This was probably due to the nature of the

Table 5.1 Reasons for having complementary treatment

	Acupuncture		Homoeopathy		Osteopathy		F Ratio	p
1 Because orthodox treatment was not effective for my particular problem.	4.51	(1.28)	4.23	(1.33)	4.48	(1.59)	0.91	ns
2 Because the orthodox treatment I received was too distressing	3.94	(2.10)	3.57	(2.16)	4.42	(2.21)	2.85	ns
3 Because the orthodox treatment I received had unpleasant side effects	4.29	(1.92)	3.80	(1.87)	4.60	(2.11)	3.03	
4 Because I believe that orthodox medicine generally has too many unpleasant side effects	3.70	(1.61)	4.24	(1.59)	4.05	(2.08)	1.96	ns
5 Because I believe that orthodox medicine is generally ineffective	3.25a	(1.72)	3.30	(1.92)	4.00	(1.87)	4.07	0.05
6 Because my doctor did not understand my problem	3.80	(1.89)	3.80	(1.93)	4.44	(1.74)	3.05	0.05
7 Because I found it difficult to talk to my doctor	3.48	(2.09)	3.71	(2.17)	4.23	(2.19)	2.58	ns
8 Because my doctor did not give me enough time	3.64a	(1.98)	4.15	(1.99)	4.42a	(1.90)	3.40	0.05
9 Because I was persuaded to come by a friend or relative	3.62	(2.02)	4.34	(2.11)	4.31	(1.72)	3.48	0.05
10 Because it was easier to get an appointment with a complementary practitioner	3.16a	(2.33)	3.62	(2.43)	4.33a	(1.89)	5.53	0.005
11 Because I have a more equal relationship with my complementary practitioner than with my doctor	3.86	(1.55)	4.18	(1.99)	4.34	(1.89)	1.52	ns
12 Because I believe complementary therapy will be more effective for my problem than orthodox medicine	4.49	(0.96)	4.50	(1.04)	4.74	(0.67)	1.98	ns
13 Because I believe that complementary medicine enables me to take a more active part in maintaining my health	4.37	(0.92)	4.69a	(0.85)	4.28a	(1.26)	3.44	0.05
14 Because I value the emphasis on treating the whole person	4.72	(0.71)	4.73	(0.87)	4.49	(1.13)	1.77	ns
15 Because I feel so relaxed after complementary treatment sessions	4.04	(1.37)	4.26	(1.76)	4.58	(1.48)	1.26	ns

	Acupuncture		Homoeopathy		Osteopathy		Mean		F ratio	sig
16 Because the explanation of my illness that I was given by my complementary practitioner made sense to me	4.06	(1.30)	4.28	(1.37)	4.42	(1.21)			1.66	ns
17 Because I value a form of therapy that involves actually touching me	3.20a	(1.72)	3.97a	(2.18)	3.58	(1.82)			3.29	0.05
18 Because I feel that complementary treatment is a more natural form of healing than orthodox medicine	3.81a	(1.40)	4.45ab	(1.030)	3.88b	(1.46)			5.44	0.001
19 Because complementary treatment is less expensive than orthodox private treatment	2.66ab	(2.04)	3.83a	(2.19)	3.63b	(2.01)			7.04	0.001
20 Because I am desperate and will try anything	3.42a	(1.97)	4.59a	(1.38)	4.01	(1.92)			8.34	0.001

Pairs of letters indicate significant differences (Scheffe comparisons)

Table 5.2 Factor scores by patient group

Factor	Acupuncture	Homoeopathy	Osteopathy	Mean	F ratio/sig
Value of complementary medicine	3.92	3.88	3.98	3.90	0.11ns
Poor doctor communication	2.85	2.95	2.89	2.90	0.19ns
Side effects or orthodox medicine	3.05a	3.01b	2.67ab	2.91	4.13 $P = 0.017$
Availability of complementary medicine	2.18a	2.37b	2.91ab	2.49	19.2 $P = 0.0001$
Orthodox medicine ineffective	3.51	3.95	3.52	3.66	7.00 $P = 0.001$

Letters indicate pairs of groups whose means are significantly different ($p < 0.05$) in Scheffe multiple comparisons.

problems they presented with and possible use of drugs by orthodox doctors. A second difference between the groups indicated that the osteopathy patients rated the availability of their therapy as more important than the other two groups. The final factor which referred to the ineffective nature of orthodox medicine was rated most highly by the homoeopathic group, who may have complaints that are particularly resistant to orthodox treatment. This would explain why group differences were no longer found after covariates, including severity of illness, were controlled for.

Other studies have failed to find marked differences between complementary medical patients and general practice patients on a range of factors: health beliefs, views on the perceived efficacy of orthodox and complementary treatments and attitudes and values (Furnham and Smith, 1988; Vincent and Furnham, 1994). Complementary medical patients do not appear to be 'in flight from science' or to have generally unusual views. Certainly some aspects of complementary therapies have a strong appeal, which is as yet insufficiently understood. A belief in the efficacy of the treatment plays a part, whether gained from personal experience or, prior to beginning treatment, from the personal recommendation of friends. This study suggests that other factors may play a part; many patients agreed that the willingness of their practitioner to discuss emotional factors, the explanation given for their illness, and the chance to play an active part in their treatment were all important reasons for seeking complementary treatment.

These programmatic studies have been part replicative and part extensional. Many of the results have been fairly consistent over different populations of complementary medicine patients. They show that general social beliefs and medical knowledge are not strong predictors of choice of practitioner. Medical history, health beliefs and their experience of practitioners are more reliable predictors of choice of complementary medicine practitioners. Further, there are very few complementary medicine patients who seek out exclusively one or more types of complementary medicine. Being both repelled and attracted by orthodox and complementary medicine at the same time, the patients appear to make a pragmatic choice of particular combinations for particular problems.

Reactions of the medical profession

Various small scale studies have been carried out in the UK to see how doctors are responding to the new climate of public interest in complementary medicine. Most have examined the attitudes of doctors, particularly general practitioners. Reilly (1983) examined the attitudes of general practitioner trainees to complementary medicine, and found that a positive attitude emerged from the 86 respondents. The majority considered acupuncture, hypnosis, homoeopathy and manipulation to be fairly useful. In all, 18 of the trainees used at least one complementary method themselves and seven wanted to train in one or more methods (especially hypnosis and manipulation). Reilly pointed out, however, that it is unlikely that general practitioner trainees are representative of the profession at large. A pilot study showed much less interest among junior hospital doctors and still less among senior doctors.

Wharton and Lewith (1986) found a high level of interest in complementary medicine among general practitioners in the UK. In total, 38% of the 145 respondents had received some training in complementary medicine and 15% wished to arrange further training. In the previous year, 76% had referred patients for alternative treatment to a doctor, 72% had referred patients to non-medically qualified practitioners and 70% thought that the more acceptable techniques, e.g. hypnosis, acupuncture, spinal manipulation and homoeopathy should be available through the National Health Service (NHS). Anderson and Anderson (1987) studied general practitioners in Oxfordshire, England and found a high level of interest in, knowledge of, and referral of patients for complementary medicine. Of the 222 respondents, 41% had attended lectures of classes in complementary medicine, 12% had received training, 42% wanted training in an alternative form of medicine, 16% were practising a form of complementary medicine and 59% had referred one or more patients to complementary medicine within the previous year.

Although the above studies were relatively small scale, they yielded comparable results, showing a generally high level of interest in complementary medicine among general practitioners. Critics of these studies have stated that many quite orthodox techniques (e.g. manipulation, counselling) were wrongly classed as complementary, so exaggerating the interest in truly complementary techniques. Visser and Peters (1990) suggested that general practitioners have a more pragmatic attitude to medicine than their hospital colleagues, which makes them more accepting of complementary medicine, although they may remain sceptical of its efficacy.

There is a considerable literature on the attitudes, beliefs, expectations and values of medical students towards various orthodox medical specialities (Furnham, 1986). In Furnham's (1986) study of medical students' attitudes to nine orthodox medical specialities, the findings showed that whereas any one speciality was perceived positively on one dimension (i.e. relationship with patients), it could also be perceived as highly negative on another (e.g. efficacy).

However, very few studies have examined medical students'

attitudes to complementary medicine. Velimirovic and Raab (1990) found that alternative medicine was popular with medical students and recent medical graduates of the University of Graz in Austria, despite the fact that the students did not know much about the theory of alternative medicine. Of these students, 69% said they would like it in their curriculum, and 63% were in favour of it being included in the National Health Service. The greatest area of doubt among the students is whether they would refer patients to an alternative practitioner outside the National Health Service; 41% said they would, while 39% were unsure. Furnham (1993) carried out a study looking at preclinical medical students' attitudes to established alternative therapies (acupuncture, herbalism, homoeopathy and osteopathy) in general and found a positive attitude among the students. Following on from Furnham's 1993 study, Furnham, Hanna and Vincent (1995) asked 180 preclinical medical students to complete one of five versions of a questionnaire concerning their attitudes to five complementary therapies: acupuncture, herbalism, homoeopathy, hypnosis and osteopathy.

These complementary therapies were chosen because they are generally well-established, well-known and definable. It was expected that the students would be a bit cautious about the therapies, but as in other studies, the results were generally positive and less hostile and negatively stereotyping than those of some practising doctors. Very few statistical differences in students' attitudes to the five therapies were found suggesting that students had similar attitudes, which were generally positive, despite the fact that they considered they knew little about the therapies.

The students all strongly agreed that they knew little about the five complementary therapies and were also uncertain about many of the attitude statements. Thus, it could be that because the students knew little or believed they knew little about the individual complementary therapies, they simply (knowingly or unknowingly) expressed their attitudes to complementary medicine in general, rather than to the particular complementary therapy they were asked about. A second possibility is that due to their lack of knowledge, the students were cautious in expressing strong beliefs about the specialities. This would have led to the many uncertain (mid-points) beliefs obtained for all the specialities. Perhaps if students were given information about the complementary specialities during their training, or if they had experience of the specialities, differences in attitudes towards them might emerge. A minority (17%) of the students had visited someone who practised complementary medicine, but almost one-third knew someone close who uses or who had used a complementary practitioner. However, this could not guarantee knowledge about the particular complementary therapy these students were questioned about. A third possibility is that because the five complementary therapies considered in the study are the more established and well-known ones, students saw them as similarly effective and beneficial. If less well-established, more controversial specialities such as faith healing, reflexology, or aromatherapy were included, the students' beliefs about them may have differed significantly from those about the more established complementary therapies.

It was interesting that male medical students were more likely than females to believe that complementary medicine is unscientific, not advancing, and that it should not be taught in medical school. Thus, male medical students seem more sceptical about complementary medicine than do females. However, it is important to remember that the correlations between sex and the attitude scales were relatively low. Also, it could just be that females were more likely to be uncertain about statements where as males were more ready to give an agree or disagree answer.

Despite their uncertainty about factors that one would expect students of orthodox medicine to take into account, such as whether or not complementary medicine has a scientific basis, and whether there is evidence for its efficacy, the students had a generally positive attitude to complementary medicine. They nevertheless believed that complementary medicine has low status in orthodox medicine, and that complementary practitioners are held in low regard by most other doctors. In all, 75% of the students believed that complementary practitioners had effective treatments, and 92% did not believe that complementary practitioners were less intelligent and less emotionally stable than other doctors. The students also recognized the holistic approach of complementary medicine, and felt that complementary practitioners spent more time listening to their patients than doctors. However, despite this, they did not believe that complementary practitioners get more satisfaction from their work than doctors. The students also agreed that a surprising number of patients claim complementary medicine is effective at curing their ills.

The students' positive attitudes to complementary medicine were, however, accompanied by caution, since 76% of the students believed there are many 'quacks' in complementary medicine. It is not, however, clear whether students believed these 'quacks' were predominantly in the established complementary therapies, in the less well-established therapies or both. The students tended to believe that all patients undergoing complementary treatment should be seen by a doctor first, and that complementary practitioners should preferably be medically qualified. They were, however, unsure about whether only doctors should practise complementary medicine.

Possibly, the students would prefer complementary practitioners to have some knowledge of or training in orthodox medicine to ensure against 'quacks' and to ensure patient safety. Though there remain relatively few studies on training or practising orthodox medical doctors, the results seem to indicate cautious acceptance rather than outright rejection of complementary medicine. This may surprise some and disappoint others, but may reflect the fact that the hubris of modern biotechnical medicine has passed its zenith.

Evidence for various hypotheses why people use and choose complementary medicine

Furnham (1994) has postulated over ten reasons why patients may choose to visit complementary practitioners. Many of these explanations are related and through examinations of the aforementioned literature, it may be possible to evaluate each.

Anti-orthodox medicine

Possible reasons that have been posited include disillusionment with the hegemony of orthodox medicine (in general) which is seen as never having reached its nineteenth century promise. Allied to this 'explanation' is the possible reason that prospective patients imbued with anti-science, anti-establishment, post-modernist theory reject 'scientific' medicine and the orthodox, positivist theory upon which it is based.

While it is possible that this explanation may be used to interpret why some people are both attracted to, but primarily flee from orthodox medicine, the above studies have revealed that this group is very small. Confined to the more articulate, educated, relatively fit middle class, theoretical or epistemological reasons do not account for much of the variance when explaining speciality choice. Further, it is possible that patients and clients develop 'theories' of their choice and rationalizations for their behaviour *post hoc*: that is, after, rather than before they made their choice.

Dissatisfaction and/or fear of orthodox professionals

There is considerably more evidence to support this type of explanation, which holds that patients of alternative practitioners have had bad experiences of orthodox doctors. These experiences come in a number of forms: first that the doctor does not seem to take the time or care to 'understand fully' the patient. That is, that patients feel they are being *processed* too quickly by the orthodox medical system. They feel cheated, possibly their expectations of a consultation are inappropriate and unreasonable; also they may be presenting with an obvious psychosomatic or trivial complaint, that busy orthodox doctors cannot deal with. Another reason for dissatisfaction lies in the patients's perception that the doctor and the cure/therapy simply does not work. That is, that their chronic condition, most frequently back pain, does not improve and that the orthodox practitioner for all the training and the advancement of modern medicine, is unable to deal with the problem.

Thirdly, there are patients who fear orthodox medical practitioners. They fear their power and their methods which some see as too technological and insufficiently sensitive to individual differences. Surgeons frequently epitomize the all-powerful, even brutal, side of medicine. Studies on health locus of control show that orthodox medical patients have more faith in their practitioner, but also take less responsibility for their own health. It really revolves around the issue of trust and the extent to which patients believe their practitioners can and do help them.

The philosophy of complementary medicine

It has been argued that some patients are attracted to specific branches of complementary medicine because of its philosophy – that is the types of explanation it gives for health and illness. This is particularly the case when explanations are both holistic and psychological. Just as people choose and read newspapers that confirm their political views, so people may seek out practitioners whose 'philosophy' fits their own. Once again while this may in part be true, it is too cognitive an explanation, particularly if people are chronically sick and seeking relief from pain.

It does not appear the case that complementary medicine patients have noticeably different health belief models compared with similar patients who are exclusive users of orthodox medicine.

Morbid self-interest and neurosis

Cynics from the orthodox medicine camp have been known to explain the behaviour of complementary patients as a manifestation of neurosis. That is, that neurotic, psychosomatic patients are drawn to the psychobabble and talking/touching cures of some complementary practitioners precisely because it is a case of psychologically disturbed people getting psychological help.

The evidence is equivocal on this point and a number of studies have shown the incidence of actual psychiatric morbidity (cases) to be higher in complementary medicine patients. Yet it could be that chronic, painful illness that appears both progressive and incurable leads to a higher incidence of neurosis and the search for alternative treatments.

Shopping for health

Few patients are exclusive users of one branch of complementary medicine. As the above studies have shown, most people have an understanding that certain types of complementary medicine are ideally suited to specific complaints, i.e. acupuncture for migraine, osteopathy for back pain, homoeopathy for allergies, etc. Equally they believe orthodox medicine to be by far the most efficient for problems associated with broken bones, bleeding, etc. The more health options available, the more people shop for health, trying out various solutions or cures to different conditions. There is more evidence that this is the case. This seems particularly true of very health-conscious people.

Conclusion

The research of the reasons for medical practitioners/speciality choice has not yielded many counterintuitive findings. However, it has failed to confirm some rather simple-minded hypotheses, such as the idea that patients of complementary medicine have totally rejected orthodox medicine; that they have alternative lifestyles or cosmologies; or that they are mentally unstable. The results show that patients shop for health; they are often disappointed by specific experiences of orthodox medicine; and that many believe they are in charge of their health.

As yet, research has not related either comprehensively the medical (or psychological) history of the patient to his or her preferred speciality. Nor has it examined specific dissatisfaction with complementary medicine practice. There is quite clearly considerably research to be done in trying to understand what are the most powerful demographic, medical, psychological and cultural predictors of why a person chooses at one particular point in their lives to consult one of the growing band of practitioners of complementary medicine.

References

Anderson, E. and Anderson, P. (1987) General practitioners and alternative medicine. *Journal of the Royal College of General Practitioners*, **37**, 52–55

Bakx, K. (1991) The 'eclipse' of folk medicine in western society. *Sociology of Health and Illness*, **13**, 17–34

Baum, M. (1989) Rationalism versus irrationalism in the care of the sick: science versus the absurd. (Editorial.) *Medical Journal of Australia*, **151**, 607–609

Bowling, A. (1994) Beliefs about illness causation among Turkish and white British people living in a deprived inner London district. *Health Education Research*, **9**, 355–364

BMA (1993) *Complementary Medicine*. Report of the Board of Science and Education. Oxford: Oxford University Press

Calnan, M. (1987) *Health and Illness*. London: Tavistock

Cant, S. and Calnan, M. (1991) On the margins of the medical marketplace? An exploratory study of alternative practitioners' perceptions. *Sociology of Health and Illness*, **13**, 34–51

Eisenberg, O., Kessler, R. and Foster, C. (1993) Unconventional medicine in the United Kingdom: patients, practitioners and consultants. *Lancet*, **ii**, 542–545

Fitzpatrick, R. (1984) Lay concepts of illness. In *The Experience of Illness*, edited by R. Fitzpatrick, J. Hinton, S. Newman, S. Scambler and J. Thompson. London: Tavistock, pp. 11–31

Fulder, S. and Munro, R. (1985) Complementary medicine in the United Kingdom: patients, practitioners and consultants. *Lancet*, **ii**, 542–545

Furnham, A. (1986) Medical students' beliefs about five different specialities. *British Medical Journal*, **293**, 1067–1680

Furnham, A. (1994) Explaining health and illness. *Social Science and Medicine*, **39**, 715–725

Furnham, A. (1993) Attitudes to alternative medicine: a study of the perception of those studying orthodox medicine. *Complementary Therapies in Medicine*, **1**, 120–126

Furnham, A. and Bhagrath, R. (1992) A comparison of health beliefs and behaviours of clients of orthodox and complementary medicine. *British Journal of Clinical Psychology*, **32**, 237–246

Furnham, A. and Forey, J. (1994) The attitudes, behaviours and beliefs of patients of conventional vs complementary (alternative) medicine. *Journal of Clinical Psychology*, **50**, 458–469

Furnham, A. and Kirkcaldy, B. (1996) The health beliefs and behaviours of orthodox and complementary medicine clients. *British Journal of Clinical Psychology*, **35**, 49–61

Furnham, A. and Smith, C. (1988) Choosing alternative medicine: a comparison of the beliefs of patients visiting a GP and a homoeopath. *Social Science and Medicine*, **26**, 685–687

Furnham, A., Hanna, D. and Vincent, C. (1995) Medical students' attitudes to complementary medical therapies. *Complementary Therapies in Medicine*, **3**, 212–219

Furnham, A., Vincent, C. and Wood, R. (1995) The health beliefs and behaviours of three groups of complementary medicine and a general practice group of patients. *Journal of Alternative Complementary Medicine*, **1**, 347–359

Lewith, C. and Aldridge, D. (1991) *Complementary medicine and the European Community*. Saffron Walden: C. W. Daniel

Moore, J., Phipps, K., Marcer, D. and Lewith, G. (1985) Why do people seek treatment by alternative medicine? *British Medical Journal*, **237**, 983–988

Reilly, D. (1983) 'Young doctors'' views on alternative medicine. *British Medical Journal,* **287**, 337–339

Research Council for Complementary Medicine (1994) *RCCM Bulletin, Number 25.* London: Research Council for Complementary Medicine

Sharma, U. (1992) *Complementary Medicine Today: Practitioners and Patients.* London: Routledge

Skrabanek, P. (1988) Paranormal health claims. *Experimentia,* **44**, 303–305

Smith, T. (1983) Alternative medicine (editorial). *British Medical Journal,* **287**, 307

ter Riet, G., Kleijnen, J. and Knipschild, P. (1990) Acupuncture and chronic pain: a criterion based meta-analysis. *Journal of Clinical Epidemiology,* **11**, 1191–99

Thomas, K., Carr, J., Westlake, L. and Williams, B. (1991) Use of non-orthodox and conventional health care in Great Britain. *British Medical Journal,* **302**, 207–210

Velimirovic, B. and Raab, S. (1990) Attitudes of medical students towards alternative medicine. *Offenthiche Gesundheitswesen,* **52**, 136–141

Vincent, C. A. and Furnham, A. (1994) The perceived efficacy of orthodox and complementary medicine. *Complementary Therapies in Medicine,* **2**, 128–134

Vincent, C. and Furnham, A. (1996) Why do patients turn to complementary medicine? An empirical study. *British Journal of Clinical Psychology,* **35**, 37–48

Vincent, C., Furnham, A. and Willsmore, M. (1995) The perceived efficacy of complementary and orthodox medicine in complementary and general practice patients. *Health Education Research,* **10**, 395–405

Visser, E. and Peters, L. (1990) Alternative medicine and general practitioners in the Netherlands: towards acceptance and integration. *Family Practitioner,* **7**, 227–232

Wharton, R. and Lewith, G. (1986) Complementary medicine and the general practitioner. *British Medical Journal,* **292**, 1498–1500.

Chapter 6

Do complementary therapies offer value for money?

Adrian R. White

Introduction

Complementary medicine has a reputation for offering value for money. Agents such as homoeopathic and some herbal remedies are relatively cheap, and an acupuncture needle costs the same as a tablet of ibuprofen 400 mg. It is often stressed by its proponents that complementary medicine uses the body's own healing force, or *vis medicatrix naturae*, which at first sight appears to be a cost-effective approach. However, complementary medicine is labour-intensive: in the UK consultations last on average 43 minutes, and courses of treatment consist of an average of 6.6 sessions (White, Resch and Ernst, unpublished data).

One population survey of 921 adults living in the UK in 1993 concluded that between 7 and 11% of the population visit practitioners of the major complementary therapies every year (Vickers, 1994). Since less than one in eight of them is dissatisfied with the treatment, it appears that about 5 million people think that complementary medicine is worth paying for (MORI, 1989). The total spending on consultations is estimated to be between £500 million and £1000 million each year. Herbal and homoeopathic remedies and aromatherapy oils worth a further £63 million were sold in 1994 (Mintel, 1995). These estimates represent an addition from private sources of 1.5–3% to the NHS annual budget of £37 billion in respect of the purchase of complementary medicine.

Homoeopathy and acupuncture are available sporadically within the NHS, but accurate figures for total purchasing are not available. Only one-third of district health authorities who responded to a survey were able to estimate their current levels of spending on complementary medicine (Cameron-Blackie and Mouncer, 1993), and the authors' estimate, that at least £1 million was spent on purchasing complementary medicine during 1991/2, is likely to be conservative. There is anecdotal evidence of increased commissioning of complementary medicine (Smith, 1995). Three-quarters of UK doctors think that some forms of complementary medicine should be available within the NHS (Perkin, Pearcy and Fraser, 1994), and other purchasers of health care, such as general practitioner fundholders and family health service authorities, are generally in favour of paying for complementary medicine, and some are already doing so (Cameron-Blackie and Mouncer, 1993).

In the USA, Eisenberg *et al.* (1993) estimated that the total expenditure on complementary medicine in 1990, including a wide selection of interventions such as commercial weight-loss programmes, amounted to approximately $13.7 billion per annum. Three-quarters of this sum was paid 'out-of-pocket' by the patient. The total sum is comparable to the $12.8 billion spent out-of-pocket annually for all hospitalizations. Fisher and Ward (1994) showed that public usage of complementary medicine is higher in all other European countries studied than in Great Britain, and sales of homoeopathic and herbal remedies are rising rapidly. In many countries complementary medicine is provided by orthodox practitioners and financed by the state.

Purchasers of health care have an ethical obligation to use state resources for the greatest good. There is an urgent need for accurate and reliable estimates of the cost-benefit of complementary medicine, as well as evidence of safety and effectiveness. Rigorous cost-evaluation studies in complementary medicine are rare. This article will review the methodology and consider some examples.

Methods of evaluation of costs of health-care

The fundamental aim of the cost-evaluation process is to measure the input of costs against the outcome of benefits, usually in order to compare two or more interventions. The methodology for the application of this process to health-care is still in the stage of development but four major methodologies have been defined (Robinson, 1993a).

Cost-minimization is the most straightforward concept. The objective is to compare the costs of different interventions which have the same finite clinical outcome. For example, a new operative technique for the repair of a hernia may be compared with a standard technique. In practice, many clinical outcomes are not single finite endpoints and *cost-effectiveness* is the appropriate procedure: its objective is to measure the costs of bringing about change in one natural outcome measure, such as the speed of functional recovery from back pain. Interventions can then be compared in terms of their costs in proportion to their effects on the outcome (e.g. manipulation versus exercise physiotherapy).

Cost-utility studies are similar in principle to cost-effectiveness studies, but measure the outcome in terms of the desirability of the intervention. This is a natural outcome though not easy to measure (see below). Society is often most interested in *cost-benefit* analysis, the objective of which is to compare the costs of an intervention with its benefits expressed in financial terms. Society will normally prefer to pay for treatments whose financial benefits exceed the costs.

Design features of cost-evaluation studies.

The basic requirements for rigour in cost-evaluation studies have been established (Coyle and Davies, 1994) and are given here: the terminology will be discussed below.

1. The question, design, and perspective must be clearly stated and appropriate.
2. The study should involve at least two alternative interventions for comparison: normally the 'do nothing', least costly and most-used options should be considered.
3. Cost information should be collected prospectively, in parallel with clinical information, in a rigorous randomized clinical trial.
4. All the relevant direct and indirect costs must be identified and assessed accurately (Table 6.1).
5. Marginal costs and benefits should be used where appropriate
6. Where estimates are made, this should be clearly stated and sensitivity analysis performed.
7. Induced costs such as the treatment of side effects must be

Table 6.1 Categories of costs required for evaluation

Direct medical costs	Service costs	Direct non-medical costs	Indirect morbidity costs	Intangible costs
Intervention costs:				
Practitioner fees	Rental of clinic rooms (or capital costs)	Transport costs	Time off work	Pain, suffering, grief
Diagnostic costs: X-rays, etc	Ancillary staff, including administrator, etc	Costs of accompanying relatives	Time off caring for family	
Therapy costs: needles, remedies, etc	Office costs including heat and light			
'Induced' costs of further treatments, including adverse reactions, must be included in the analysis				

included, and the time-scale of the study must permit their identification.

8. Discounting must be performed, so that future costs and benefits are assessed in today's values.
9. Close scrutiny of cost-variations should be performed
10. Methods used should be transparent, and reports of the study should be comprehensive so that it can be understood and reproduced.

Measuring costs

The perspective of the evaluation must be established at the outset as it is critical in determining which costs need to be measured. For example a new treatment for back pain might involve additional costs from the NHS perspective, but might save the nation as a whole considerable sums in terms of sickness benefit and lost production. The conclusions of research into economic effectiveness may have financial consequences and bias in funding this research is a real risk (Task Force Report, 1995). Every effort should be made to avoid bias in design, performance and reporting; leading journals now require that sources of funding and potential conflicts of interest are declared by the authors (*Lancet*, 1993).

Costs should be estimated prospectively, with clinical data; studies which estimate costs retrospectively are inferior. Larger sample sizes may be required for cost-evaluation analysis than for effectiveness-only studies since cost measurements are not subject to inclusion and exclusion criteria and therefore are liable to show greater variation than clinical outcomes.

Complementary medicine has features which may require particular attention when measuring costs. First, practitioner fees should include a component for reimbursement of the considerable costs of self-funded training; tuition fees at the British School of Osteopathy, for instance, are currently £22 000. Second, complementary medicine often involves long consultations and repeated attendances, and direct non-medical costs such as travel and time off work are likely to have a significant effect on the result of the study. These costs are difficult to measure and 'shadow pricing' is justified, in which average values are used, for example for the effect of time lost from work (Robinson, 1993b). Third, complementary medicine is widely perceived as safe, but complications do occur and the time-span of the trial must permit these to be identified; costs of treating complications should be included under 'induced costs'.

Opportunity costs should strictly speaking be used for staff and equipment, i.e. the cost of their next most efficient use if they were not employed in the study. However, actual market costs are adequate in most cases. It is usually appropriate to measure the marginal costs and benefits which represent expansion or contraction at the margins of a service that is already provided. Marginal costs are generally lower than average costs, e.g. the daily costs of inpatient treatment fall with the duration of the admission, and average costs would overestimate the effect of early discharge.

When treatment costs are likely to continue for more than one year, it is recommended that calculations should discount future costs to present day values by a factor of 6% per annum. This process recognizes that costs incurred in the near future appear more important than those in the distant future, and reflects the rate of inflation and the effect of interest (Robinson, 1993b). There is still discussion as to whether discounting should also apply to benefits on the basis that patients would prefer benefits sooner rather than later.

Utility and quality-of-life

The concept of 'utility' was first formulated as a test of an act's public or private morality, i.e. whether it promoted the 'greatest happiness' of the greatest number of people. It is clear that greatest happiness involves a full assessment of quality of life and covers a wide range of dimensions (a dimension is an area of interest which is measured by several interrelated variables, e.g. mental state is a dimension measured by cognitive level, mood, affect etc). In health care the appropriate measurement is health-related quality of life, and Robinson (1993a) defined utility as 'the subjective level of well-being that people experience in different states of health'.

It has been noted that complementary medicine practitioners claim that benefits of complementary medicine such as well-being are non-specific and rather intangible, that its effectiveness is underestimated if all that is measured is change in symptoms, and that patient acceptability of the therapy itself should be included (Mercer et al., 1995). It is likely that subjective health-related quality of life will be an appropriate outcome measure for complementary medicine.

The ideal quality of life measure for cost-utility studies would yield a single global figure so that all diseases and treatments can be compared and priorities established. The Rosser matrix aims to do this by using trained observers to rate health status in two dimensions, disability and distress. This establishes a figure on a scale of 1 (no health problems) to 0 (dead). The method has been shown to be reliable, although not particularly comprehensive; an alternative is the Euroqol questionnaire which probably lacks sensitivity (Fitzpatrick,

1994). The life-expectancy can be multiplied by the index to calculate the quality adjusted life year (QALY). The costs per quality adjusted life year of various interventions can be ranked into a league table as a guide for purchasing health care (Mason, Drummond and Torrance, 1993). This process has limitations and potential sources of inaccuracy, but life-expectancy is not normally influenced by complementary medicine, and other methods will be more appropriate.

Quality-of-life measures for use as clinical outcomes need to strike a balance between being simple and standardized, so that they can operate across different diseases and treatments, and subtle and individual so that they genuinely reflect the subject's own view. Self-administered questionnaires have a clear cost advantage over those that require an interview. Each instrument has been developed for a specific target group such as sufferers from cancer, or rheumatoid arthritis, or a healthy population, and should only be used within the area of its demonstrated validity (Gill and Feinstein, 1994). Recent questionnaires have concentrated on combining brevity with precision and are likely to encourage a high response rate (Ware, 1993). Two general purpose instruments are widely used in the UK. The Nottingham Health Profile (part one; the second part is rarely used) contains 38 items which measure six dimensions (pain, physical mobility, energy, emotions, sleep, social contacts) and was originally conceived as a population survey tool (Jenkinson, Fitzpatrick and Argyle, 1988). It can provide a valid and reliable picture of health status, but it has certain problems. Questions were designed to be answered dichotomously (yes/no) so that it was easier to complete, but respondents may find this restricting. Each dimension is designed to be weighted according to a predefined scoring system, but Jenkinson (1994) showed that this adds little to the accuracy and a great deal to the complexity.

The Short-Form 36 (SF-36) contains 36 questions which yield scores in eight dimensions in the three main areas of functional status, well-being and overall evaluation of health. It can be completed in about 10 minutes, and has been demonstrated to possess internal consistency, test-retest reliability, and construct validity (Brazier *et al.* 1992). It is more sensitive to lower perceived levels of ill-health than the Nottingham Health Profile, which is important for research in complementary medicine. It is not yet established how accurately the SF-36 can detect changes over time or different populations, nor how meaningful any detected changes are. Two other potential difficulties are that it was not designed to be used for economic modelling, so its relevance for this purpose has not been validated; and it was not designed to yield a single global figure for quality of life.

The problem of accurately reflecting the patient's viewpoint is addressed more directly by the schedule for the evaluation of individual Quality of life (SEIQoL). Respondents are first assisted in choosing from a list the five dimensions which they deem most important for their quality of life, and they then respond to questions which assess the impact of the illness in these five areas (McGee *et al.*, 1991). This technique has the disadvantage of relying on interviews.

This cumulative evidence implies that the SF-36 is the most appropriate current instrument for complementary medicine, but it should be combined with specific validated disease-related measures (Cox *et al.*, 1992).

Formal cost-evaluation studies have been performed in orthodox medicine (e.g. Gerard, 1991; Coyle and Davies, 1993) but few are available in complementary medicine. Some studies include a retrospective estimate of costs and benefits and will now be discussed in order to illustrate the methods and suggest possible fruitful areas for further research.

Examples of cost-minimization analysis

Generic herbal preparations may be cheaper than modern drugs with the same indication. For instance, *Crataegus* could be compared with ACE inhibitors for heart failure, or *Hypericum* with selective serotonin reuptake inhibitors in mild/moderate depression, since these are two herbal remedies whose effectiveness has been established (Weihmayr and Ernst, 1995; Ernst, 1995). Acupuncture in combination with ondansetron may reduce the required dosage of this expensive drug for the satisfactory control of nausea postoperatively or during chemotherapy. No formal comparisons are available.

Herbal extracts containing β-sitosterol are routinely prescribed for benign prostatic hypertrophy in mainland Europe, whereas in the UK a transurethral resection is more usual. A double-blind, randomized, controlled trial recently compared the effect of β-sitosterol with placebo in 200 subjects (Berges *et al.*, 1995). The results showed a significant improvement in Boyarsky score, urinary flow, voiding time and residual urine volume, in favour of the treatment group. Once effectiveness has been demonstrated for a treatment, the evaluation of its costs becomes relevant.

Using a cost-minimization exercise, the costs of β-sitosterol and transurethral resection can be compared. Costs for supervision and prescription were added to the purchase price of the drug; and estimates were made of the cost of consultation at either 2-monthly or 6-monthly intervals, at £35 per attendance. Figures were also obtained for costs of transurethral resection in the South-West of England, and three values were selected representing the lowest (£808), the highest (private hospital, £2695) and most-used (general practitioner fundholder charge, £1330). Other consultation costs and the costs of investigation were assumed to be equal in the two cases. Costs of future treatment were discounted at 6% per annum, and calculated annually for the first 5 years, and for 10 years. Induced treatment costs of side effects were also estimated: β-sitosterol has no recorded side effects, whereas transurethral resection results in an estimated 5–10% readmission rate for repeat surgery. Estimates were made using both figures. Direct non-medical costs associated with treatment, and indirect costs were excluded on the assumption that they are similar in the two groups. No allowance was made for differing rates of patient satisfaction resulting from the two procedures. Sensitivity analysis was performed on the range of estimates for different consultation rates and different re-operation rates (Table 6.2).

The results demonstrate the critical influence that follow-up consultation rates may have on the evaluation. A general practitioner fundholder minimizes costs over 10 years by prescribing β-sitosterol if 6-monthly follow up is clinically sufficient. The conclusions of this exercise are obviously subject to the prevailing local costs.

Cost-effectiveness and cost-utility analyses

One trial will be used to illustrate the principles of these methods since it suggests the possibility of significant economies in stroke rehabilitation. Johansson et al. (1993) described an open controlled study of acupuncture in patients with recent stroke. Seventy-eight

Table 6.2 A sensitivity analysis showing cumulative costs (£) per patient of β-sitosterol treatment, at low and high rates of follow up consultation; compared with cost of transurethral resection in three hospitals, and two different rates of readmission (see text)

Year	1	2	3	4	5	10
β-sitosterol 6-monthly consultation	300	508	702	878	1042	1165
β-sitosterol 2-monthly consultation	650	992	1312	1602	1874	2077
				5% readmission	10% readmission	
Transurethral resection	Lowest price NHS hospital			848	899	
	Cost to general practitioner fundholder			1397	1463	
	Private hospital			2830	2965	

patients with recent hemiparesis were randomized either to receive 20 sessions of acupuncture, or to act as no-treatment controls. Both groups received daily physiotherapy and occupational therapy. The duration of stay in hospital and Nottingham Health Profile scores at one year were measured. The trial was designed as a clinical study and not a cost-evaluation analysis, so the costs of acupuncture treatment were not actually measured.

Cost-effectiveness depends on the assessment of an appropriate natural outcome, in this case duration of stay in hospital. This appears rigorous as the research team were not involved in the decision to discharge the patients. The results show that the acupuncture group's inpatient stay was approximately half the control group's (87 days instead of 166 days). Approximately 90% of the acupuncture group had been discharged home at one year, compared with 70% of the controls ($P < 0.02$, chi-square). If treatment costs had been measured it would be a simple matter to calculate the costs per day of reduced inpatient care. One criticism of this study is that the treatment group received considerable attention which was not controlled for, and the results of placebo-controlled studies should be awaited before any conclusions can be drawn about the cost-effectiveness of acupuncture in stroke.

The same study also provided information about the quality of life via the Nottingham Health Profile, which would be appropriate for a cost-utility analysis. The intervention group scored significantly higher (i.e. improvement) for mobility and emotional problems (30 and 9 respectively) than the no-treatment control group (49 and 28 respectively; $P < 0.05$). Scores for other dimensions of the profile showed trends in favour of the intervention, but did not reach significance.

Cost-benefit analysis

Cost-benefit analysis balances the financial benefits of treatment against its costs. The perspective of the person asking the question will determine which costs are included. For example, figures from Johansson's same study can be used to demonstrate a cost-benefit analysis from the point of view of the hospital and residential home costs. The decreased use of nursing home and rehabilitation facilities was estimated to have reduced the mean direct cost by $26 000 per patient in the treatment group. It was not stated whether marginal costs were used, which would be correct. From society's perspective, this saving in hospital costs will be partially balanced by the extra costs of community care for the discharged patients. From the patients' perspective, there will be a negative cost-benefit in financial terms but this will be offset by the intangible benefit of being home earlier.

Another open controlled trial in which retrospective (and therefore limited) estimates of cost-benefit were made was described by Christensen *et al.* (1992). Twenty-nine patients were recruited from the waiting-list for knee replacement surgery to receive acupuncture. A second group served as waiting-list controls before they too received acupuncture.

Twenty-two patients showed significant improvements in various objective scores for pain and mobility. Those who responded continued to receive monthly acupuncture treatment, and seven patients gained sufficient pain relief to remove themselves from the waiting-list for surgery (follow-up period 49 weeks). The total estimated saving in operating costs was $63 000. No measurement was made of the cost of the 310 treatments given, nor the costs of future treatment or the non-medical or indirect costs.

Hospital inpatients have psychological needs and when these are met by appropriate services earlier discharge can be achieved (House, Farthinc and Peveler, 1995). Nurses and other staff are making increasing use of aromatherapy and massage; aromatherapy with peppermint oil was shown to relax muscles and improve mood (Gobel, Schmidt and Soyka, 1994), and neroli oil may have medium-term benefits, although its short-term effect is insignificant (Stevensen, 1994). A controlled trial of massage showed benefit in depression (Ernst and Fialka, 1994) although the contribution of non-specific factors was not excluded. Opportunity costs will need to be carefully assessed before the adoption of these procedures can be supported. These reports do not supply sufficient data for rigorous cost-evaluation analyses and further studies are required.

Cost-benefit in primary care

To what extent does the introduction of one (or more) complementary therapies affect the expenditure of the practice? Swayne (1992) analysed computerized prescription records and showed that 22 homoeopathic general practitioners working within the NHS issued 12% fewer prescriptions than the average for their area. The net mean ingredient cost was 20p less than average. The author pointed out the limitations of this study, which did not compare defined groups of patients and measured outcomes with control groups. Dixon (1995) measured prescribing costs of 50 chronic patients who received healing, and found that savings of £1500 more than offset the healer's expenses of £950. Peters, Davies and Pietroni (1994) measured referral rates to physiotherapy and rheumatology from their general practice which runs its own musculoskeletal clinic, and found them to be below the national average. Such studies may not have compared like with like and randomized clinical trials are needed for proper evaluation.

Feldhaus (1993) reviewed the incidence of postoperative complications of dental surgery for one year before and 7 years after prescribing *Arnica montana 12X* routinely at the time of surgery. The complication rate fell to 40% below the average for other dentists in the region. There are several possible explanations for this finding, such as alterations in dental technique, skills of auxiliary personnel etc, but this is an important claim and a suitable subject for a double-blind, randomized, controlled trial.

The general principles for such cost-benefit studies with the purchaser's perspective are as follows: costs must be measured for fixed duration before and after the introduction of the therapy. A control purchaser or group must be recruited, matched as closely as possible for staff and patient profile, drug costs, referral rates, and facilities. The control must make no relevant changes in practice which would affect costs. Such cost-benefit studies should not of course ignore clinical outcomes when the effectiveness of the test therapy has not been demonstrated.

Cost evaluation of complementary medicine in back pain treatment

One promising area where complementary medicine may be cost-beneficial to society and to individuals is the treatment of back pain. The prevalence of back pain in the UK has remained relatively constant but there has been an large increase in disability (CSAG Report, 1994). It is estimated that 10–20% of the workforce lost time from work through back pain in 1993, contributing to a national total of a loss of over 100 million workdays. Half of this number is caused by acute back pain, and half by pain lasting more than 4 weeks. Surveys show that 3–4% of people aged 16–44 years and 5–7% of those aged 45-64 years report back pain as 'chronic sickness'. Back pain costs the NHS approximately £0.5 billion per annum in treatment, but costs the nation about ten times as much, consisting of £1.4 billion in social security payments, and an estimated £4 billion in lost production.

The Clinical Services Advisory Group (CSAG) has identified two major targets for cost-benefit, i.e. rehabilitating acute back pain sufferers and preventing the progression to chronic pain. It was calculated that increasing the use of active rehabilitation and manipulation could improve outcomes by the order of 30–50%, and that the costs of this could be offset by reduced need for analgesics and hospital admissions, and by other recommendations which include a policy of reduction in the use of X-rays.

Stano (1993) used a novel method to compare the costs of chiropractic and orthodox medical care for back pain in the USA. Computerized records were obtained for all payments made by health insurance companies over a 2-year period (some 400 000 cases) in respect of back pain treatment. Insurance payouts for patients using orthodox medical care were approximately $1000 higher per case than for chiropractic care. The additional cost was entirely due to inpatient care, mainly surgery; outpatient attendances for orthodox care were fewer and cheaper than for chiropractic care. There are recognized limitations with the use of claims databases such as coding inaccuracies, limited amount of clinical information, and socio-economic differences between groups with restrictions on insurance cover. A later study (Stano 1994) included corrections for these features, and the result was essentially the same. However, there remain two major drawbacks to this approach, i.e. that the patients who present for chiropractic or orthodox medical care may not have equal severity of back pain, and there is no comparison of outcomes. Therefore the author does not appear to be justified in his conclusions that chiropractic treatment minimizes the costs of back pain management.

A pragmatic controlled trial of low back pain treatment was conducted by Meade *et al.* (1990, 1995) in which 781 subjects without contraindications to manipulation were randomized to receive either chiropractic or standard NHS outpatient management of low back pain. The main endpoint was the Oswestry score measured by means of a self-administered questionnaire, with a maximum of 100. Initial mean Oswestry scores were approximately 30 points in both groups, and improved after 2 years to about 10 (chiropractic) and 17 (outpatients), a significant difference. After 3 years the difference was less marked at 3.18 (95% confidence interval 0.16–6.20) but still statistically significant. Other outcome measures including straight-leg raising and lumbar flexion showed parallel changes. The residual 3-year difference between groups is also clinically significant, representing a change from moderate pain to no pain, or the ability to sit for one hour instead of half an hour.

Figures for treatment costs were given and a cost-evaluation can be performed. The average cost of chiropractic investigation and treatment at 1988–9 prices was £165 per patient compared with £111 for hospital treatment. The cost-effectiveness per percentage point on the Oswestry score after 2 years was therefore £9.70 for chiropractic and £11.10 for hospital outpatients; but after 3 years the cost-effectiveness was reversed at £11.70 for chiropractic and £10.18

for hospital outpatients; this calculation has not taken into account (because figures are not available) the fact that 42% of the chiropractic group received extra treatment during the 3 years, but only 31% of the hospital group did.

Approximately 72 000 UK patients per annum were estimated by Meade *et al.* (1990) to have no contraindication to chiropractic, and if all those received chiropractic within the NHS instead of outpatient treatment there would be an increase in marginal direct treatment costs of £4 million. The outcome of the trial suggested that chiropractic would result in an average annual reduction in work loss of 2 days per patient treated, which the authors calculated would save in the region of £8 million in the first year in output and social security payments.

Meade's study compared settings not therapies and does not provide evidence in support of the effectiveness of manipulation itself, and in fact 72% of the outpatient group received Maitland mobilization or manipulation. It is recognized that the result may also have been influenced by factors such as the different atmosphere of an unhurried private chiropractic consultation compared with a typical NHS outpatients clinic, and the high motivation of the chiropractors who instigated the study.

Several meta-analyses of the effect of manipulation in the treatment of acute back pain have been performed (e.g. Koes *et al.*, 1991; Shekelle *et al.*, 1992). The balance of opinion is that the evidence is strongly suggestive of a specific effect, but not conclusive. Shekelle *et al.* combined the data and applied a Heyes probability procedure to calculate that manipulation resulted in an increase of between 0.11 and 0.17 in the probability of recovery at 2–3 weeks. This represents an improvement in the recovery rate at this point from 50% to 67%.

The benefit of manipulation is likely to be short-lived because of the high remission rate in untreated cases. Most studies with adequate follow-up periods show no difference at 12 months. However, a clinical study by Koes *et al.* (1992), published after these meta-analyses, compared the effect of manipulation, physiotherapy, placebo and general practitioner treatment of low back pain. Manipulation was slightly superior to physiotherapy in improving back pain after 12 months, and both treatments were significantly better than either placebo or general practice management.

A cost-evaluation of back pain management has recently been published (Carey *et al.* 1995). Two hundred and eight practitioners involved in primary care of back pain were randomly selected from professional registers. They comprised primary care physicians, chiropractors, orthopaedic surgeons and nurse practitioners/physician's assistants from a health maintenance organization. They recruited

1633 consecutive patients who presented with untreated back pain of less than 10 weeks' duration. Subjects were assessed prospectively by research staff, and their progress was followed over the next 6 months. Direct treatment costs were estimated with reference to average state-wide charges for each provider for the investigation and treatment given. No other costs were measured or estimated.

Results showed that there was no difference between the groups in time to functional recovery, return to work or complete recovery. Median treatment costs per case were significantly higher for management by orthopaedic surgeon ($383) and urban chiropractic ($545) than for urban primary care ($169) or health maintenance organization provider ($184). This was mainly accounted for by increased use of magnetic resonance imaging and physiotherapy by the orthopaedic surgeons, and by the increased number of attendances and use of radiology by the chiropractors. Use of medications was significantly lower and patient satisfaction significantly higher among the patients treated by chiropractors than in all other groups.

This trial examined the pragmatic situation with practitioners chosen at random rather than for their special research interest, and it may therefore reflect the situation in everyday clinical practice more accurately than some other studies. The strength of the study is compromised by the lack of observers blinding to the intervention, and lack of patient randomization.

Conclusion

There is no hard evidence to support the notion that complementary medicine is cost-beneficial, and further trials are necessary. Herbal medicine appears to afford the possibility of competing with orthodox care for certain indications. There is only weak evidence of cost-benefit for homoeopathy in dental care, and for acupuncture in stroke and arthritis. The efficacy of manipulation in acute back pain has some support but its effectiveness in practice has been questioned. The methodology of cost-evaluation is established and rigorous trials should be designed, although some problems remain with the assessment of quality of life.

References

Berges, R. R., Windeler, J., Trampisch, H. J. and Senge, Th. (1995) Randomised, placebo-controlled, double-blind clinical trial of β-sitosterol in patients with benign prostatic hyperplasia. *Lancet*, **i**, 1529–1532

Brazier, J. E., Harper, R., Jones, N. M. B., O'Catnain, A., Thomas, K. J., Usherwood, T. et al. (1992) Validating the SF-36 health survey questionnaire: new outcome measure for primary care. British Medical Journal, 305, 160–164

Cameron-Blackie, G. and Mouncer, Y. (1993) Complementary therapies in the NHS. Research Paper 10, NAHAT, Birmingham Research Park, Vincent Drive, Birmingham B15 2SQ

Carey, T. S., Garrett, J., Jackman, A., McLaughlin, C., Fryer, J., Smucker, D. R. et al. (1995) The outcomes and costs of care for acute low back pain among patients seen by primary care practitioners, chiropractors, and orthopedic surgeons. New England Journal of Medicine, 333, 913-917

Cox, D. R., Fitzpatrick, R., Fletcher, A. E., Gore, S. M., Spiegelhalter, D. J., Jones, D. R. et al. (1992) Quality-of-life assessment: can we keep it simple? Journal of the Royal Statistical Society, 155, 353–393

Christensen, B. V., Iuhl, I. U., Vilbek, H., Bulow, H. H., Dreijer, N. C., Rasmussen, H. F. et al. (1992) Acupuncture treatment of severe knee osteoarthrosis. A long-term study. Acta Anaesthetica Scandinavica, 36, 519-525

Coyle, D. and Davies, L. (1994) How to assess cost-effectiveness: elements of a sound economic evaluation. In: Purchasing and Providing Cost-effective Health care, (edited by M. F. Drummond and A. Maynard). Edinburgh: Churchill Livingstone. pp. 66–79

CSAG Committee Report (1994) Back Pain. London: HMSO

Dixon, M. (1995) A healer in the practice. British Journal of General Practice, 45, 6

Eisenberg, D. M., Kessler, R. C., Foster, C., Norlock, F. E., Calkins, D. R., Delbanco, T. L. et al. (1993) Unconventional medicine in the United States. New England Journal of Medicine 328, 246–252

Ernst, E. (1995) St John's Wort as an antidepressant? A systematic criteria-based review. Phytomedicine, 2, 67–71

Ernst, E. and Fialka, V. (1994) Clinical effectiveness of massage therapy – a critical review. Forschende Komplementarmedizin, 1, 226–232

Feldhaus, H-W. (1993) Cost-effectiveness of homoeopathic treatment in a dental practice. British Homoeopathic Journal, 82, 22–28

Fisher, P. and Ward, A. (1994) Complementary medicine in Europe. British Medical Journal, 309, 107–111

Fitzpatrick, R. (1994) Applications of health status measures. In: Measuring Health Outcomes, edited by C. Jenkinson. London: UCL Press

Gerard, K. A. (1991) Review of cost-utility studies: assessing their policy-making relevance. HERU discussion paper 11/91. Aberdeen: Department of Public Health and Economics, University of Aberdeen

Gill, T. M. and Feinstein, A. R. (1994) A critical appraisal of the quality of quality-of-life measurements. Journal of the American Medical Association, 272, 619–626

Gobel, H., Schmidt, G. and Soyka, D. (1994) Effect of peppermint and eucalyptus oil preparations on neurophysiological and experimental algesimetric headache parameters. Cephalalgia, 14, 228–34

House, A., Farthinc, M. and Peveler, R. (1995) Psychological care of medical patients (Leader). British Medical Journal, 310, 1422–1423

International Committee of Medical Journal Authors (1993) Conflict of interest (Editorial). Lancet, i, 742–743

Jenkinson, C., Fitzpatrick, R. and Argyle, M. (1988) The Nottingham Health Profile: an analysis of its sensitivity in differentiating illness groups. Social Science Medicine, 27, 1411–1414

Jenkinson, C. (1994) Weighting for ill-health: the Nottingham Health Profile. In:

Measuring Health and Medical Outcomes, (edited by C. Jenkinson). London: UCL Press. pp. 77–88

Johansson, K., Lindgren, I., Widner, H., Wiklund, I. and Johansson, B. B. (1993) Can sensory stimulation improve the functional outcome in stroke patients? *Neurology*, **43**, 2189–2192

Koes, B. W., Assendelft, W. J. J., van der Heijden, G. J. M. G., Bouter, L. M. and Knipschild, P. G. (1991) Spinal manipulation and mobilisation for back and neck pain: a blinded review. *British Medical Journal*, **303**, 1298–1303

Koes, B. W., Bouter, L. M., van Mameren, H., Essers, A. H. M., Verstegen, G. M. J. R., Hofhuizen, D. M. *et al.* (1992) Randomised clinical trial of manipulative therapy and physiotherapy for persistent back and neck complaints: results of one year follow-up. *British Medical Journal*, **304**, 601–605

McGee, H. M., O'Boyle, C. A., Hickey, A., O'Malleya, K. and Joyce, C. R. B. (1991) Assessing the quality of life of the individual: the SEIQoL with a healthy and a gastroenterology unit population. *Psychological Medicine*, **21**, 749–759

Mason, J., Drummond, M. and Torrance, G. (1993) Some guidelines on the use of cost-effectiveness tables. *British Medical Journal*, **306**, 570–572

Meade, T. W., Dyer, S., Browne, W., Townsend, J. and Frank, A. O. (1990) Low back pain of mechanical origin: randomised comparison of chiropractic and hospital outpatient treatment. *British Medical Journal*, **300**, 1431–1437

Meade, T. W., Dyer, S., Browne, W. and Frank, A. O. (1995) Randomised comparison of chiropractic and hospital outpatients management for low back pain: results from extended follow up. *British Medical Journal*, **311**, 349–351

Mercer, G., Long, A. F. and Smith, I. J. (1995) *Researching and evaluating complementary therapies: the state of the debate.* A report for Nuffield Institutes of Health, University of Leeds

Mintel Intelligence Report. (1995) *Complementary Medicines.* Mintel, 18-19 Long Lane, London EC1A 9HE

MORI. (1989) *Alternative Medicine Survey.* London: MORI

Perkin, M. R., Pearcy, R. M. and Fraser, J. S. (1994) A comparison of the attitudes shown by general practitioners, hospital doctors and medical students towards alternative medicine. *Journal of the Royal Society of Medicine*, **87**, 523–525

Peters, D., Davies, P. and Pietroni, P. (1994) Musculoskeletal clinic in general practice: study of one year's referrals. *British Journal of General Practice*, **44**, 25–29

Robinson, R. (1993a) Economic evaluation and health care: what does it mean? *British Medical Journal*, **307**, 670–673

Robinson, R. (1993b) Costs and cost-minimisation analysis. *British Medical Journal*, **307**, 726–728

Shekelle, P. G., Adams, A. H., Chassin, M. R. *et al.* (1992) Spinal manipulation for low-back pain. *Annals of Internal Medicine*, **117**, 590–597

Smith, I. (1995) Commissioning complementary medicine. *British Medical Journal*, **310**, 1151–1152

Stano, M. (1993) The economic role of chiropractic: an episode analysis of relative insurance costs for low back care. *Journal of the Neuromusculoskeletal System*, **1**, 64–68

Stano, M. (1994) Further analysis of health care costs for chiropractic and medical patients. *Journal of Manipulative and Physiological Therapeutics*, **17**, 442–446

Stevensen, C. J. (1994) The psychophysiological effects of aromatherapy massage following cardiac surgery. *Complementary Therapy in Medicine*, **2**, 27–35

Swayne, J. (1992) The cost and effectiveness of homoeopathy. *British Homoeopathic Journal*, **81**, 148–150

Task Force Report. (1995) Economic analysis of health care technology: a report on principles. *Annals of Internal Medicine*, **122**, 6170

Vickers, A. (1994) Use of complementary therapies (Letter). *British Medical Journal*, **309**, 1161

Ware, J. E. (1993) Measuring patients' views: the optimum outcome measure (Editorial). *British Medical Journal*, **306**, 1429–1430

Weihmayr, Th. and Ernst, E. (1995) Die therapeutische Wirksamkeit von Crataegus. *Fortschritte der Medizin*, **1–2**, 27–9

Chapter 7

The use and abuse of evidence-based medicine: an example from general practice

George T. Lewith

Introduction

The practical utilization of clinical trial data raises a number of important issues in the context of general practice. First, and probably the most obvious, is that many clinicians tend to read clinical trials in a relatively uncritical manner so consequently may use the limited information inappropriately, if indeed they use it at all. The relevance and applicability of clinical trial literature is therefore dependent on the reader's education and ability to evaluate evidence. Predigested information, such as that produced by meta-analysis or the Cochrane collaboration is often difficult to access in the context of general practice.

Much of the early information published in the field of complementary medicine was grossly inadequate; for instance many researchers assumed that sham acupuncture was in fact a placebo, so naturally came to rather inappropriate conclusions about the use of acupuncture. These were based on their inadequate understanding of the field and the consequently inadequate trial methodology that was applied in order to answer their poorly thought-through questions (Lewith and Machin, 1983).

It has long been recognized that the more rigorous a clinical trial, potentially the less it may be generalized. Pragmatic studies such as those produced by Meade *et al.* (1990) may in many ways be more open to generalization, but are prone to major criticisms because of their lack of rigour. As Oxman (1994) has suggested, there are no 'magic bullets' and treatment advantages are often small and difficult to measure.

Risk-benefit ratios are another difficult issue. They involve the clinician and patient, in partnership, balancing the effects of an effective invasive procedure, which may have a high chance of adverse reaction, against a non-invasive, possibly less effective but much safer approach to the same problem. The balance of benefit versus harm will vary from clinician to clinician and patient to patient, often providing problems if we attempt to suggest that an idealized treatment exists for a particular condition.

An implicit assumption within evidence-based medicine is that it will provide us with much harder data upon which to decide how to manage patients; in a recent article in the *Lancet*, Rothwell (1995) suggested that while clinical trials may be applicable to some patients, and could provide guidelines as to how they should be managed, the fundamental assumptions which underpin the application of clinical trial results to clinical practice, particularly general practice, have rarely, if ever, been tested. Do our research-based conclusions operate in the same way in a clinical environment? All too often we select an unusual group of patients for clinical trials for whom it may be impossible to apply the same treatment criteria as we do on a day-to-day basis in clinical practice. Consequently, the very pragmatic and simple nature of outcome studies may provide us with more information about the costs, benefits, risks and outcomes of treatments as they are actually applied in day-to-day clinical medicine.

The evidence base

In spite of these more general problems that are associated with the field of complementary therapies, an evidence base for complementary medicine is beginning to emerge. Lewith and Vincent (1995) have analysed the information in relation to acupuncture in a critical manner and suggested new strategies for the development of clinical trials. On balance, it would appear that there is some evidence to suggest that acupuncture is of value in a variety of painful conditions (Lewith and Vincent, 1995), as a mechanism for smoking withdrawal and, last but not least, in the treatment of nausea (Vickers, 1994). Meade *et al.* (1990) have shown that in spite of the inherent problems that exist within pragmatic clinical trials, chiropractic provided in a private practice environment (as compared to physiotherapy provided in an NHS environment) is effective in the management of chronic low back pain in both the short and long term. Koes *et al.* (1991) have also demonstrated the value of manipulation in low back pain and neck pain. Reilly *et al.* (1994), in their recent article in the *Lancet*, also argue powerfully that homoeopathy has an effect greater than that expected from purely placebo medication, again providing evidence that homoeopathy may be doing something when utilizing the model of homoeopathic immunotherapy in asthma and hay fever. While none of these areas can individually be seen as a great breakthrough for complementary medicine, they represent small building blocks in that they provide some degree of evidence which argues cogently for the use of these techniques.

It is no longer either valid or reasonable for physicians to suggest that there is no evidence within complementary medicine. The fact that it is sometimes conflicting and unclear in many ways places the diverse disciplines comprising complementary medicine on the same level as many areas within conventional medical management. No-one would argue with a suggestion that more research is needed, but perhaps it may be pertinent to ask how much research and how much difference will it make? However much evidence we have about manipulation and back pain, general practitioners will still refer polysymptomatic patients to the osteopath working in their practice for management of their back pain. These patients represent an entirely different population, quite possibly with a different illness, to those entered into large clinical trials. The only similarity is that both groups of patients have back pain. It is evident that a large proportion of these referrals are inappropriate for the osteopath acting as a biomechanical physician and all too often would be excluded from a clinical trial, but they nevertheless represent a treatment option that the general practitioner finds useful and the patient beneficial (Peters, Davies and Pietroni, 1994). What use are rigorous clinical trials in this situation when the general practitioner simply wishes to find a harmless treatment option so that the patient is sympathetically handled and cared for.

Implementation

In spite of the fact that good evidence is available which undoubtedly supports the use of complementary medicine in one or two areas, the evidence is far from being implemented in clinical practice. Again, complementary medicine shows many parallels with conventional medicine; research is all too often ignored and that which is widely quoted, often misinterpreted. Until we can develop a better evidence-based system with associated implementation guidelines throughout the National Health Service, it is unlikely that we will find our approach to evidence-based medicine becoming implemented. Without implementation, we will never discover whether our evidence base is valid in clinical practice.

For instance, Koes *et al.* (1991) and Meade *et al.* (1990) provide powerful evidence that manipulation is effective in the context of back pain in general practice. Meade's pragmatic study compares private chiropractic practice with a variable assortment of NHS physiotherapy practice. Koes's data are much more rigorous. When, however, we come to look at how the principle is implemented in general practice, an entirely different picture emerges. Peters, Davies and Pietroni (1994) show clearly that general practitioners refer polysymptomatic patients who may have back pain into osteopathic services. Such referrals have no evidence base, but it may be that data relevant to therapeutic touch rather than manipulation are important for these individuals. These three papers question, at a fundamental level, the value of randomized controlled trials in the management of the polysymptomatic patient in general practice (Meade *et al.*, 1990; Koes *et al.*, 1991; Peters, Davies and Pietroni, 1994).

The consultation

Charlton (1993) has suggested that probably the most important part of medical intervention is the holistic and humane doctor. He presents an idealized environment in which the doctor is wise, compassionate, liberally educated, part-time and supremely well informed. An ideal to which we would all wish to adhere but in essence may be somewhat impractical. Cousins (1988) has continued to emphasize, in many of his publications, the importance of psychoneuroimmunology and the effect that a whole variety of unmeasured and possibly unmeasurable psychological factors have both in the consultation and in recovery from illness. He emphasizes the importance of the patient-physician interaction quoting the view of medical thinkers down the centuries, including Holmes, Osler and Bernard. He suggests that the physician has a prime resource at his disposal in the form of the patient's own apothecary, particularly when this is combined with a prescription pad. In a recent article in the *Lancet*, Thomas (1994), concludes that the placebo effect in general practice is the power of the doctor alone to make the patient feel better, irrespective of the medication provided. He goes on to argue that this, probably the most important factor in any consultation, is generally neglected, unrecognized and untaught. In view of these observations, often supported by hard evidence (Thomas 1987), how can we believe in evidence-based medicine solely grounded on the randomized, placebo-controlled trial?

Conclusion

The literature would suggest, contrary to some popular belief, that complementary medicine does have some disciplined methodology within the field of clinical trials. In spite of under-funding and methodological inadequacies, a balance of positive evidence for the use of complementary medicine is emerging. However, it is, and always will be, difficult to interpret realistically any clinical trial evidence from primary care in the context of the patient-doctor relationship and to understand how this interaction will affect outcome, whether the treatment is of proven effectiveness or questionable benefit. In the context of these arguments, it is probably fair to conclude that evidence-based medicine and the use of clinical trials alone will always be of limited value in clinical practice. Perhaps, in this context, patient demand for complementary therapies may be both a powerful and clinically valuable asset.

Complementary medicine has a number of important cross-cultural aspects. The disease and treatment models that are applied raise fundamental questions about the construction involved in 'clinical reality' (Kleinman, Eisenberg and Good, 1978). So even if we can demonstrate that a particular therapeutic approach has fundamental validity in one culture, will it be applicable cross-culturally?

The only conclusion that we can draw from these diverse and conflicting arguments may well be that we need a variety of different mechanisms for evaluating particular therapeutic interventions which include an assessment of the patient's relationship with the doctor, uncontrolled evaluations of particular therapeutic interventions, singularly or in combination, rigorous clinical trial evidence, an assessment of the patient's belief system and, last, but not least, an understanding of the cultural context in which the treatment will be provided.

References

Charlton, B. (1993) Holistic medicine or the humane doctor? *British Journal of General Practice*, **43**, 475–477

Cousins, N. (1988) Intangibles in medicine; an attempt at a balancing perspective. *Journal of the American Medical Association*, **250**, 1610–1612

Kleinman, A., Eisenberg, L. and Good, B. (1978) Clinical lessons from anthropologic and cross cultural research. *Annals of Internal Medicine*, **36**, 251–258

Koes, B., Assendelft, W., Van der Heijden, G., Bouter, L. and Knipschild, P. (1991) Spinal manipulation and mobilisation for back and neck pain; a blinded review. *British Medical Journal*, **303**, 1298–1303

Lewith, G. and Machin, D. (1983) On the evaluation of the clinical effects of acupuncture. *Pain*, **16**, 111–127

Lewith, G. and Vincent, C. (1995) Evaluation of the clinical effects of acupuncture: a problem re-assessed and a framework for future research. *Pain Forum*, **4**, 29–39

Meade, T., Dyer, S., Browne, W., Townsend, J. and Frank, A. (1990) Low back pain of mechanical origin; randomised comparison of chiropractic and hospital outpatient treatment. *British Medical Journal*, **300**, 1431–1437

Oxman, A. (1994) No magic bullets. A systematic review of 102 trials of intervention as to how health care professionals deliver services more effectively or efficiently.

Prepared for the North East Regional Thames Authority, March 1944

Peters, D., Davies, P. and Pietronni, P. (1994) Musculoskeletal clinic in general practice – a study of one year's referrals. *British Journal of General Practice*, **44**, 25–29

Reilly, D., Taylor, M., Beattie, G., Campbell, J., McSharry, C., Aitchison, T. *et al.* (1994) Is evidence for homoeopathy reproducible? *Lancet*, **ii**, 1610–1616

Rothwell, P. (1995) Can overall results of clinical trials be applied to patients? *Lancet*, **i**, 1616–1618

Thomas, K. B. (1987) General practice consultations: is there any point in being positive? *British Medical Journal*, **294**, 1200–1202

Thomas, K. B. (1994) The placebo in general practice. *Lancet*, **ii**, 1066–1067

Vickers, A. (1994) P6 acupuncture point stimulation as an anti-emetic therapy. A report commissioned by North East Thames Regional Health Authority.

Chapter 8

Direct risks associated with complementary therapies

Edzard Ernst

Introduction

Adverse reactions to medical interventions have recently received much attention (e.g. Kahn, 1995; Rawlins, 1995). It is estimated that about 4% of all hospitalized patients suffer from adverse reactions, that in the USA approximately 180 000 individuals die each year from adverse reactions and that in the ambulatory setting this costs $77 billion per year (Bates, Cullen and Laird, 1995; Johnson and Bootman, 1995).

While the general public becomes more and more aware of adverse reactions to orthodox therapies, complementary treatments are perceived as natural and hence devoid of adverse reactions. In fact, one important reason for turning towards complementary options is the expectation to be helped without the risk of adverse reactions (e.g. Ernst, Willoughby and Weihmayr, 1995).

Unfortunately, the notion that natural can be equated with harmless is at best misleading, at worse it is dangerously wrong. The following discussion will focus on *direct* adverse reactions associated with some of the most prevalent complementary therapies, homoeopathy, phytomedicine (herbalism), acupuncture and spinal manipulation. Chapter 9 will detail the *indirect* risks that may be encountered in complementary medicine.

Homoeopathy

'Homoeopathy is . . . a non-toxic system of medicine' (Chopra, 1994). Quotes to this effect can be found in virtually every book on the subject. Opponents of homoeopathy claim that it has no effect at all, therapeutic or otherwise (Kerr and Saryan, 1986). But is this assumption really true?

Even if one assumes that homoeopathy remedies are pure placebos, one has to consider that such treatments do induce adverse reactions

Table 8.1 Nocebo effects according to frequency

Headache
Drowsiness
Tiredness
Dizziness
Nausea
Pain
Insomnia

Overall incidence = 19% (pooled data from 109 studies)

According to Rozenzweig Petal, *Clinical Pharmacology and Therapeutics* 1993, **54**, 578.

in the form of nocebo effects (De Smet, 1992). Table 8.1 lists the most common nocebo effects. These are usually mild and benign and therefore represent no serious safety issue.

Yet the literature also reports serious adverse reactions of homoeopathy. After repeated dilution, varying concentrations of the original substance can still remain. Potentially toxic concentrations of arsenic (Kerr and Saryan, 1986) and cadmium (De Smet, 1992) have been found in homoeopathic preparations, and one case of an acute pancreatitis following the administration of a complex homoeopathic remedy (Kerr, 1986) has been reported. Low potency preparations can also cause allergic reactions; several such reports have been published (e.g. Van Ulsen, Stolz and Joost, 1988; Forsman, 1991). In view of such findings interactions with other treatments are conceivable in concomitant drug treatments, although there is no published evidence for or against this occurring.

An interesting peculiarity of homoeopathy is that, according to the homoeopathic literature, 'aggravations' of the conditions under treatment can occur. If they do, homoeopaths view this as confirmation that the chosen remedy was correct. The question whether these homoeopathic aggravations are a real phenomenon or whether they are merely a reflection of the natural course of the disease has not been addressed systematically. Should homoeopathic aggravations be real, they would need to be considered as a possible adverse reaction of homoeopathic therapy.

Generally speaking adverse reactions to homoeopathic medication are probably rare. Yet the fact is that we cannot, at present, tell their true incidence as no definitive study to establish the facts has ever been carried out. Under-reporting in mainstream medicine is huge, with only about 5–10% of all adverse reactions being reported (Rawlins, 1995). Under-reporting in homoeopathy, or indeed any other form of complementary medicine, is an unknown entity. There is little reason to assume that it is less than in conventional medicine.

Phytomedicine (herbalism)

During the last few years, adverse reactions to herbal preparations have received increasing attention (e.g. Atherton, 1994; Harper, 1994). Several authoritative texts on the subject have been published (e.g. D'Arcy, 1991; Hänsel, R. *et al.*, 1992; De Smet, 1994a), and the literature on this topic is vast. Therefore only very recent (1994) contributions will be cited as *examples* of direct adverse reactions to herbal remedies.

Allergic reactions

Herbal preparations can, of course, lead to hypersensitivity. Reports of reactions abound (e.g. Li, Zhao and Li, 1994; Lin and Ho, 1994), and these can vary from dermatitis to anaphylactic shock. For instance, tea tree oil (melaleuca oil), widely used as a topical disinfectant, or camomile can cause allergic reactions (Knight and Hausen, 1994; Bossuyt and Dooms-Goossens, 1994).

Toxic reactions

Adverse reactions like severe nephropathy (Lin and Ho, 1994) and colitis (Beaugerie, Luboinski and Brusse, 1994) have been associated with flavonoids which are contained in most plants. The ingestion of valerian root, skullcap and chaparral as a tea has been associated with acute hepatitis (Caldwell *et al.*, 1994) confirming earlier suspicions of liver toxicity of (some of) these plants.

Momordica charantia is an anti-diabetic herb also used as a common vegetable in Sri Lanka; its fruit juice contains hepatotoxins (Tennekoon *et al.*, 1994). Thorn apple tea has been reported to cause anticholinergic adverse reactions (Coremans *et al.*, 1994). The squirting cucumber (*Ecbalium elaterium*) is used as a purgative; a case of cardiac and renal failure has been associated with its use (Vlachos and Kanitsakis, 1994). Sassafras and germander have also been repeatedly shown to be hepatotoxic (De Smet, 1994a; Loeper *et al.*, 1994).

Traditional eye medicines have been reviewed elsewhere (Harries and Cullinan, 1994); in some African countries their use is associated with 25% of corneal ulcers and 26% of childhood blindness. In Tanzania 58% of patients with corneal ulcers had no other plausible cause of ulceration than the use of local traditional remedies (Yorston and Forster, 1994).

Chinese herbal preparations have been associated with renal fibrosis and renal failure. These followed the administration of a slimming drug containing aristolochic acid (Vanhaelen *et al.*, 1994); more than 30 women died. Seven cases of acute hepatitis have been reported following a Chinese herbal sedative and analgesic that apparently has been in traditional use for more than 1000 years (Woolf *et al.*, 1994). A further case of hepatitis was reported; this time the cause was possibly *Cortex dictamni radicis* (Pillans, Eade and Massey, 1994).

One case of pneumonia after the intake of the Japanese traditional medicine 'Saiboku-To' has also been reported. The patient was successfully treated and took the remedy again which resulted in a recurrence of pneumonia (Temaru *et al.*, 1994).

Mutagenic reactions

Anthranoid laxatives like aloe, cascara, rhubarb and senna have genotoxic potential in several test systems, and have been associated with colorectal cancer in epidemiological studies in humans. Some national authorities have therefore imposed restrictions (Anonymous, 1994). Further and different studies are required to clarify this important issue.

Betel nut quid contains alkaloids which can form nitrosamines in the saliva. It has been implicated in the development of oral cancer (Pickwell, Schimelpfening and Palinkas, 1994).

Chaparral may also be mutagenic. One case has been described where a patient developed cystic renal cell carcinoma after regularly drinking chaparral tea (Smith *et al.*, 1994).

Other adverse effects

Additional adverse reactions have been noted in the medical literature. While they are, in the main, isolated reports of unknown significance, they nevertheless illustrate the need for vigilance.

- Smoking ginseng cigarettes has been associated with a general deterioration of mental functions in schizophrenic patients (Wilkie and Cordess, 1994). Discontinuation of this habit resulted in clinical improvement.
- *Agnus castus*, taken during an unstimulated cycle, showed considerable derangement of gonadotrophin and ovarian hormone levels (Cahill *et al.*, 1994) in a woman undergoing in-vitro fertilization. *Agnus castus* may therefore lead to ovarian hyper-stimulation and may increase the risk of miscarriage.
- Many plants contain salicylates rendering salicylism a potential risk of herbal treatments. One case of salicylism with vomiting and

generalized seizures has been described (Malik, Zabidi and Noor, 1994). The child had accidentally swallowed 20 ml of a traditional remedy containing oil of wintergreen, camphor, peppermint, menthol and oil of eucalyptus.

- Khat chewing is popular in Arabian countries. *Catha edulis* contains the amphetamine-like compound cathinone. It can have euphorigenic effects and lead to sympathicomimetic adverse reactions (Widler *et al.*, 1994).
- Yohimbine has α_2-adreno receptor antagonist properties. Bronchospasm and a lupus-like syndrome have been reported (De Smet and Smeets, 1994).

Drug interactions

Interactions of phytomedicines with concomitantly administered prescription drugs is another under-researched issue. Both an enforcement or an enhancement of activity are conceivable. The ingestion of grapefruit juice, for instance, elevates serum concentrations of cyclosporin, calcium-channel blockers and other drugs by competing competition for the same metabolic pathway (Bailey, Arnold and Spence, 1994).

Contamination

Ayurvedic medicines use arsenic and other highly toxic substances as ingredients. Mercury, lead and other heavy metal contamination may occur due to the peculiar manufacturing process of these remedies (Keen *et al.*, 1994).

Several Chinese herbal remedies have been demonstrated to be adulterated by undeclared prescription medicines. Adverse reactions including acute interstitial nephritis have been described (Diamond and Pallone, 1994). Chinese herbal preparations for systemic or topical use may contain powerful steroids (Hughes, Higgins and Pembroke, 1994). Self-prescribed use during 1 month led to a Cushing-like syndrome that was reversible after drug discontinuation (Stricht *et al.*, 1994). There have also been cases of lead poisoning due to contaminated Chinese herbal medicines (Markowitz *et al.*, 1994).

False authentication

False authentication can, of course, happen inadvertently or deliberately. An example of the former is the outbreak of fibrosing

interstitial nephritis in Germany and France following the administration of a slimming aid. In these preparations the Chinese drug
'Fangji' was substituted by 'Guang fangji' containing nephrotoxic
aristolochic acids (Arzneimittelkommission, 1994; Pourrat, Montastrue and Lacombe, 1994). In another case, a medication did not
contain, as declared, the aphrodisiac yohimbine but caffeine (De Smet
and Smeets, 1994). Ginseng preparations are also problematic in this
respect (Cui et al., 1994). Only Asian ginseng contains ginsenosides,
the active compounds, but commercial preparations often do not make
this clear.

Acupuncture

While the discussion as to the efficacy of acupuncture continues (e.g.
Patel et al., 1989; ter Riet, Kleijnen and Knipschild, 1990), adverse
reactions associated with its use are being reported.

Risk of infection

If acupuncture needles are to be re-used they require adequate
sterilization. When one way material is employed, it requires adequate
handling to guarantee sterility. If such basic safety rules are not
strictly adhered to, there is a high risk of transmitting infections.

Several case reports exist in which acupuncture was the only
plausible explanation for an infection with HIV (Castro et al., 1988;
Vittecoq et al., 1989). Hepatitis B and C infections have also been
transmitted in this way (e.g. Boxall, 1978; Kent et al., 1988;
Mitchitaka, Horiike and Ohta, 1991). One epidemiological study from
Japan identified acupuncture to be a risk factor for hepatitis C
infections (Kiyosawa, Tanaka and Sodeyama, 1994). A recent review
on the subject (Rampes and James, 1995) identified 126 cases of
acupuncture-related hepatitis in the world literature. Others have
reported that osteomyelitis (Jones and Cross, 1980), endocarditis,
peritonitis (Rampes and James, 1995) and generalized Staphylococcus
aureus infections (Baltimore and Moloy, 1976) have been transmitted
through the use of acupuncture needles. One author has mentioned
cellulitis following acupuncture (Peacher, 1975). It can be assumed
that all blood-borne infections are transmittable through the (mis)-use
of acupuncture needles.

Trauma

By definition, acupuncture needles cause tissue trauma. If the technique is performed properly, only the skin and the connective tissue below will be affected. If, however, acupuncture needles are inserted at the wrong site or penetrate too deeply, other tissues or organs can be damaged.

Several cases of pneumothorax and haemothorax have been documented (Ritter and Tarala, 1978; Wright, Kupperman and Liebhaber, 1991; Gray, Maharajh and Hyland, 1991; Norheim and Fonnebo, 1995). Peacher also mentioned injury of the middle ear (after auriculoacupuncture) and to the spinal cord (Peacher, 1975). Cardiac tamponade has been another, potentially fatal traumatic complication (Gray, Maharajh and Hyland, 1991). A recent report describes one such event with a fatal outcome (Halvorsen *et al.*, 1995).

Needles may also break while *in situ*, particularly if the acupuncture therapy entails mechanical (manual) stimulation of the needle. Parts of acupuncture needles have been found in patients' organs and structures, e.g. kidney (Cheng, 1991), carpal tunnel (Keller, Palmer and Garvin, 1972), cervical spine (Southworth and Hartwig, 1990), spinal cord (Murata *et al.*, 1990), heart (Shiraishi *et al.*, 1979), peritoneal cavity, stomach, liver and transverse colon (Gerard, Wilke and Schiano, 1995).

If a blood vessel is punctured, haematomas may ensue; this could prove to be more than a transient cosmetic problem. Petechiae and other forms of bleeding have also been reported following acupuncture (Peacher, 1975). If a nerve is punctured the patient might experience unnecessary pain and sustain minor or, in extreme cases, persistent nerve damage. Focal myopathic changes may result from intramuscular insertion of acupuncture needles (Peacher, 1975).

Other problems

Allergies following acupuncture have been described (Hasegawa *et al.*, 1991); if the allergen in the needle is known the problem can be avoided through the proper choice of needles. Eisenberg observed several cases of 'acupuncture addiction' in China (Eisenberg, 1985). Chiu warned that acupuncture in pregnant women might carry a risk for the fetus by increasing oxytocin release in the mother (Chiu, 1984). Convulsions, inadvertent anaesthesia, loss of coordination and tinnitus have also been reported (Peacher, 1975), and aggravation of pre-existing symptoms could be a problem (Peacher, 1975). Finally, skin melanoma (Chiu, 1984) and Koebner phenomenon (Tsukerman, 1970) have been described. Table 8.2 summarizes adverse reactions other than those caused by trauma or infection.

Table 8.2 Adverse reactions to acupuncture (other than infections or traumatic)

Condition	Number of cases reported
Angina pectoris	1
Compartment syndrome	1
Contact dermatitis	5
Drowsiness	79
Epileptic seizure	1
Erythema	4
Excessive sweating	1
Fainting	142
Granuloma	2
Herpes zoster reactivation	1
Increased pain	58
Insomnia	1
Koebner phenomenon	1
Lymphoedema	2
Malaise	1
Menstruation disturbance	3
Nausea/vomiting	25
Psychiatric disorders	20
Syncope	53

Pooled data from Rampes and James, 1995 and Norheim and Fonnebo, 1995.

Spinal manipulation

Vascular accidents

The most frequent complications of manipulation of the spine are vascular accidents. The Stroke Council of the American Heart Association registered 359 such cases until 1981 (Robertson, 1981). In Switzerland, 1255 incidents were recorded in 1 535 000 manipulations (Dvorakj, 1983). Others estimated its incidence to be 1–4 per million treatments (Hosek *et al.*, 1981; Gutmann, 1983; Hamann *et al.*, 1993). Recently a group of 177 Californian neurologists reported 55 strokes associated with spinal manipulation within a 2-year period (Lee *et al.*, 1995). The mortality/severe long-term impairment rate of such events has been reported to be 28% (Frisoni and Anzola, 1991).

The incidence rate is higher if minor symptoms are included and specifically searched for: out of a total of 75 500 procedures applied, 25 such cases were reported (Michaeli, 1991). Any reported incidence rates are likely to be underestimations of the true figures. In a series of 13 cases of clinically and radiologically verified vertebral artery dissection, eight were spontaneous, two occurred after manipulation and three after minor injury (Mas *et al.*, 1987).

The pathogenetic mechanisms of vascular complications involve vertebral artery dissection, intramural bleeding or pseudoaneurysm leading to thrombosis or embolism (Frisoni and Anzola, 1991) as well as temporary interruption of blood flow through mechanical compression during cervical rotation (Green and Joynt, 1959) and vasospasm (Smith and Estridge, 1962). The vertebral artery at the C_1/C_2 segment is most often affected. Combined rotation, extension and traction movements apparently create the highest risk, particularly when executed forcefully (Stevens, 1985). Thus responsible manipulators aim at avoiding such interventions.

The most frequent clinical findings are Wallenberg's (28%), other brain stem (49%), cerebellar (8%), occipital lobe (5%) and unclassified syndromes (Frisoni and Anzola, 1991). They occur usually during or shortly after the intervention, but delays of hours, even days have also been observed (Okawara and Nibbelink, 1974; Frumkin and Baloh, 1990; Lee et al., 1995). Initially symptoms are often non-specific; headache and neck pain are the most common. Interestingly, such symptoms are frequent reasons for applying manipulative therapies in the first place. At least one case has been described where neck pain was the first sign of dissection, which in turn was treated by manipulation and in turn caused a fatal stroke (Mas et al., 1989). Others have pointed out that as many as half of the complications of manipulative treatments develop after more than one therapeutic session (Frisoni and Anzola, 1991).

Other complications

Dislocations and fractures of vertebrae have also been reported (Schmitt, 1988; Halderman and Rubinstein, 1992). Fractures seem to be rare. Patients with osteoporosis are, however, at a relatively high risk. Manipulation is therefore contraindicated in these individuals. Nerve lesions range from plexus paralysis and ophthalmoplegia to tetraplegia, disc herniation and phrenic nerve palsy (Schmitt, 1988; Tolge, Iyer and McConnell, 1993). Neurological complications seem to be less frequent. A recent review reported 89 such cases in the English language literature (Tolge, Iyer and McConnell, 1993).

Conclusions

Complementary treatments are clearly *not* free of risks. At present our data are insufficient to give exact prevalence figures. This area therefore deserves to be studied systematically. In addition to direct risks, these therapies are associated with indirect risks which are detailed in Chapter 9.

References

Anonymous. (1994) Anthranoid-haltige Humanarzneimittel. *Pharmaceutische Zeitung*, **133**, 2791–2794

Arzneimittelkommission der Deutschen Apotheker. (1994) Chinesisches Pflanzenpulver. *Deutsch Apotheker Zeitung*, **134**, 2212

Atherton, D. (1994) Towards the safer use of traditional remedies. *British Medical Journal*, **308**, 673–674

Bailey, D. G., Arnold, J. M. O. and Spence, J. D. (1994) Grapefruit juice and drugs – how significant is the interaction? *Clinical Pharmcokinetics*, **26**, 91–98

Baltimore, R. S. and Moloy, P. J. (1976) Perichondritis of the ear as a complication of acupuncture. *Archives of Otolaryngology*, **102**, 572–573

Bates, D. W., Cullen, D. J. and Laird, N. (1995) Incidence of adverse drug events and potential adverse drug events. *Journal of the American Medical Association*, **274**, 29–34

Beaugerie, L., Luboinski, J. and Brusse, N. (1994) Drug induced lymphocytic colitis. *Gut*, **35**, 426–428

Bossuyt, L. and Dooms-Goossens, A. (1994) Contact sensitivity to nettles and camomile in 'alternative' remedies. *Contact Dermatitis*, **31**, 131–132

Boxall, E. H. (1978) Acupuncture hepatitis in the West Midlands. *Journal of Medical Virology*, **2**, 377–379

Cahill, D. J., Fox, R., Wardle, P. G. and Harlow, C. R. (1994) Multiple follicular development associated with herbal medicine. *Human Reproduction*, **9**, 1469–1470

Caldwell, S. H., Feeley, J. W., Wieboldt, Th. F., Featherston, P. L. and Dickson, R. C. (1994) Acute hepatitis with use of over-the-counter herbal remedies. *Virginia Medical Quarterly*, **121**, 31–33

Castro, K. G., Lifson, A. R., White, C. R., Bush, T. J., Chamberland, M. E., Lekatsas, A. M. and Jaffe, H. W. (1988) Investigations of AIDS patients with no previously identified risk factors. *Journal of the American Medical Association*, **259**, 1338–1342

Cheng, T. O. (1991) Pericardial effusion from self-inserted needle in the heart. *European Heart Journal*, **12**, 958

Chiu, D. T. (1984) The use of acupuncture during pregnancy. *International Journal of Medicine*, **1**, 19–21

Chopra, D. (1994) *Alternative Medicine, the Definitive Guide*. Puyallup Washington: Future Medicine. p. 272

Coremans, P., Lambrecht, G., Schepens, P., Vanwelden, J. and Verhaegen, H. (1994) Anticholinergic intoxication with commercially available thorn apple tea. *Clinical Toxicology*, **32**, 589–592

Cui, J., Garle, M., Eneroth, P. and Björkhem, I. (1994) What do commercial ginseng preparations contain? *Lancet*, **ii**, 134

D'Arcy, P. F. (1991) Adverse reactions and interactions with herbal medicines. Part 1, Adverse Reactions. *Toxicology Review*, **10**, 189–208

De Smet, P. A. G. M. (1992) Giftige metalen in homeopathische preparaten. *Pharmaceutische Weekblatt*, **127**, 125–126

De Smet, P. A. G. M. (1994a) *Adverse Effects of Herbal Drugs*. Berlin: Springer Verlag

De Smet, P. A. G. M. (1994b) Een alternatieve die met een luchtje. *Pharmaceutische Weekblatt*, **129**, 258

De Smet, P. A. G. M. and Smeets, O. S. N. M. (1994) Potential risks of health food products containing yohimbe extracts. *British Medical Journal*, **309**, 958

Diamond, J. and Pallone, Th. L. (1994) Acute interstitial nephritis following use of Tung Shueh pills. *American Journal of Kidney Disease*, **24**, 219–221

Dvorakj, J. (1983) *Manuelle Medizin*. Stuttgart: Thieme

Eisenberg, D. (1985) *Encounters with Qi. Exploring Chinese Medicine*. New York: W. W. Norton and Co. pp. 118–119

Ernst, E., Willoughby, M. and Weihmayr, T. H. (1995) Nine possible reasons for choosing complementary medicine. *Perfusion*, **8**, 356–358

Forsman, S. (1991) Homeopati kan vara farling vid hudsjukdomar och allergier. *Läkartidningen*, **88**, 1672

Frisoni, G. B. and Anzola, G. P. (1991) Vertebrobasilar ischemia after neck motion. *Stroke*, **22**, 1452–1460

Frumkin, L. R. and Baloh, R. W. (1990) Wallenberg's syndrome following neck manipulation. *Neurology*, **40**, 611–615

Gerard, P. S., Wilke, E. and Schiano, Th. (1995) Images in clinical medicine: acupuncture needle fragments. *New England Journal of Medicine*, **332**, 1792

Graham-Brown, R. A., Bourke, J. F. and Bumphrey, G. (1994) Chinese herbal remedies may contain steroids. *British Medical Journal*, **308**, 473

Gray, R., Maharajh, G. S. and Hyland, R. (1991) Pneumothorax resulting from acupuncture. *Canadian Association of Radiology Journal*, **42**, 139–140

Green, D. and Joynt, R. J. (1959) Vascular accidents to the brain stem with neck manipulation. *Journal of the American Medical Association*, **170**, 522–524

Gutmann, G. (1983) Injuries to the vertebral artery caused by manual therapy. *Mannuelle Therapie*, **21**, 2–14

Halderman, S. and Rubinstein, S. M. (1992) Compression fractures in patients undergoing spinal manipulative therapy. *Journal of Manipulative and Physiological Therapeutics*, **15**, 45–54

Halvorsen, T. B., Anda, S. S., Naess, A. B. and Levang, O. W. (1995) Fatal cardiac tamponade after acupuncture through congenital sternal foramen. *Lancet*, **i**, 1175

Hamann, G., Felber, S., Haass, A., Strittmatter, M., Kujat, C., Schimrigk, K. *et al.* (1993) Cervicocephalic artery dissection due to chiropractic manipulations. *Lancet*, **i**, 764–765

Hänsel, R., Keller, K., Rimpler, H. and Schneider, G. (eds) (1992) *Hager's Handbuch der Pharmazeutischen Praxis*, vols 4–6. Berlin: Springer Verlag

Harper, J. (1994) Traditional Chinese medicine for eczema. *British Medical Journal*, **308**, 489

Harries, A. D. and Cullinan, T. (1994) Herbis et orbis: The dangers of traditional eye medicines. *Lancet*, **i**, 1588

Hasegawa, J., Noguchi, N., Yamasaki, J., Kotake, H., Mashiba, H., Sasaki, S. *et al.* (1991) Delayed cardiac tamponade and hemothorax induced by an acupuncture needle. *Cardiology*, **78**, 58–63

Hosek, R. S., Schram, S. B., Silverman, H., Myers, J. B. and Williams, S. E. (1981) Cervical manipulation. *Journal of the American Medical Association*, **245**, 922–925

Hughes, J. R., Higgins, E. M. and Pembroke, A. C. (1994) Oral dexamethasone masquerading as a Chinese herbal remedy. *British Journal of Dermatology*, **130**, 261

Johnson, J. A. and Bootman, J. L. (1995) Drug-related morbidity and mortality. *Archives of Internal Medicine*, **155**, 1949–1956

Jones, R. D. and Cross, G. III. (1980) Suspected chronic osteomyelitis secondary to acupuncture treatment. *Journal of the American Podiatry Association*, **70**, 149–151

Kahn, K. L. (1995) Above all, do no harm. *Journal of the American Medical Association*, **274**, 75–76

Keen, R. W., Deacon, A. C., Delves, H. T., Moreton, J. A. and Frost, P. G. (1994) Indian herbal remedies for diabetes as a cause of lead poisoning. *Postgraduate Medical Journal*, **70**, 113–114

Keller, W. J., Palmer, S. G. and Garvin, J. P. (1972) Possible renal complications of acupuncture. *Journal of the American Medical Association*, **222**, 1559

Kent, G. P., Brondum, J., Keenlyside, R. A., Lafazia, L. M. and Scott, H. D. (1988) A large outbreak of acupuncture-associated hepatitis B. *American Journal of Epidemiology*, **127**, 591–598

Kerr, H. D. (1986) Pancreatitis following ingestion of a homeopathic preparation. *New England Journal of Medicine*, **314**, 1642–1643

Kerr, H. D. and Saryan, L. A. (1986) Arsenic content of homoeopathic medicines. *Clinical Toxicology*, **24**, 451–459

Kiyosawa, K., Tanaka, E. and Sodeyama, T. (1994) Transmission of hepatitis C in an isolated area in Japan. *Gastroenterology*, **106**, 1596–1602

Knight, T. E. and Hausen, B. M. (1994) Melaleuca oil (tea tree oil) dermatitis. *Journal of the American Academy of Dermatology*, **30**, 423–427

Lee, Ph. K., Carlini, W. G., McCormick, G. F. and Albers, G. W. (1995) Neurologic complications following chiropractic manipulation. *Neurology*, **5**, 1213–1215

Li, L.-F., Zhao, J. and Li, S.-Y. (1994) Exanthematous drug eruption due to Chinese herbal medicines. *Contact Dermatitis*, **30**, 252–253

Lin, J. L. and Ho, Y. S. (1994) Flavonoid-induced acute nephropathy. *American Journal of Kidney Disease*, **23**, 433–440

Loeper, J., Descatoire, V., Letteron, P., Moulis, C., Degott, C., Dansette, P. *et al.* (1994) Hepatotoxicity of germander in mice. *Gastroenterology*, **106**, 464–472

Malik, A. S., Zabidi, M. H. and Noor, A. R. (1994) Acute salicylism due to accidental ingestion of a traditional medicine. *Singapore Medical Journal*, **35**, 215–216

Markowitz, S. B., Nunez, C. M., Klitzman, S., Munski, A. A., Kim, W. S., Eisinger, J, et al, (1994) Lead poisoning due to Hai Ge Fen. *Journal of the American Medical Association*, **271**, 932–934

Mas, J. L., Bousser, M. G., Hasboun, D. and Laplane, D. (1987) Extracranial vertebral artery dissections – a review of 13 cases. *Stroke*, **18**, 1037–1047

Mas, J. L., Henin, D., Bousser, M. G., Chain, F. and Haw, J. J. (1989) Dissecting aneurysm of the vertebral artery and cervical manipulation: a case report with autopsy. *Neurology*, **39**, 512–515

Michaeli, A. (1991) Dizziness testing of the cervical spine: can complications of manipulations be prevented? *Physiotherapy Theory and Practice*, **7**, 243–250

Mitchitaka, K., Horiike, N. and Ohta, Y. (1991) An epidemiological study of hepatitis C virus infection in a local district in Japan. *Rinsho Bvori*, **39**, 586–591

Murata, K., Nishio, A., Nishikawa, M., Ohinata, Y., Sakaguchi, M. and Nishimura, S. (1990) Subarachnoid haemorrhage and spinal root injury caused by acupuncture needle-case report. *Neurology in Medicine and Surgery*, **30**, 956–959

Norheim, A. J. and Fonnebo, V. (1995) Adverse effects of acupuncture. *Lancet*, **345**, 1576.

Okawara, S. and Nibbelink, D. (1974) Vertebral artery occlusion following hyperextension and rotation of the head. *Stroke*, **5**, 640 642

Patel, M., Gutzwiller, F., Paccaud, F. and Marazzi, A. (1989) A meta-analysis of acupuncture for chronic pain. *International Journal of Epidemiology*, **18**, 900–906

Peacher, W. C. (1975) Adverse reactions, contraindications and complications of acupuncture and moxibustion. *American Journal of Chinese Medicine*, **3**, 35–46

Pickwell, S. M., Schimelpfening, S. and Palinkas, L. A. (1994) 'Betelmania'. Betel quid chewing by Cambodian women in the United States and its potential health effects. *Western Journal of Medicine*, **160**, 326–330

Pillans, P. I., Eade, M. N. and Massey, R. J. (1994) Herbal medicine and toxic hepatitis. *New Zealand Medical Journal*, October, **107**, 432–433

Pourrat, J., Montastrue, J. L. and Lacombe, J. L. (1994) Néphropathie associée des herbes chinoises. 2 cas. *Presse Medicale*, **23**, 1669

Rampes, H. and James, R. (1995) Complications of acupuncture. *Acupuncture and Medicine*, **13**, 26–33

Rawlins, M. D. (1995) Pharmacovigilance. *Journal of the Royal College of Physicians*, **29**, 41–49

Ritter, H. G. and Tarala, R. (1978) Pneumothorax after acupuncture. *British Medical Journal*, **2**, 602–603

Robertson, J. F. (1981) Neck manipulation as a cause of stroke. *Stroke*, **12**, 1

Scheel, O., Sundsfjord, A., Lunde, P. and Anderson, B. M. (1992) Endocarditis after acupuncture and injection-treatment by a natural healer. *Journal of the American Medical Association*, **267**, 56

Schmitt, H. P. (1988) Risiken und Komplikationen der Manualtherapie der Wirbelsäule aus neuralogischer Sicht. *Nervenarzt*, **59**, 32–35

Shiraishi, S., Kuroiwa, Y., Nishio, S. and Kinoshita, S. (1979) Spinal cord injury as a complication of acupuncture. *Neurology*, **29**, 1188–1190

Smith, A. Y., Feddersen, R. M., Gardner, K. D. Jr, Davis, C. J. Jr (1994) Cystic renal cell carcinoma and acquired renal cystic disease associated with consumption of chaparral tea: a case report. *Journal of Urology*, **152**, 2089–2091

Smith, R. A. and Estridge, M. N. (1962) Neurologic complications of head and neck manipulations. *Journal of the American Medical Association*, **182**, 528–31

Southworth, S. R. and Hartwig, R. H. (1990) A complication of acupuncture. *Journal of Hand Surgery*, **15**, 111–112

Stevens, A. J. J. E. (1985) Zur Dopplersonographie der A. vertebralis bei Rotation des Kopfes. In: *Arteria vertebralis. Traumatologie und funktionelle Pathologie*, edited by G. Gutman. Berlin: Springer Verlag. pp. 90–99

Stricht, B. V., Parvais, O. E., Vanhaelen-Fastré, R. J. and Vanhaelen, M. H. (1994) Remedies may contain cocktail of active drugs. *British Medical Journal*, **308**, 1162

Temari, R., Yamashita, N., Matsui, S., Ohta, T., Kawasaki, A. and Kobayash, M. (1994) A case of drug induced pneumonitis caused by Saiboku-To. *Japanese Journal of Thoracic Diseases*, **32**, 485–490

Tennekoon, K. H., Jeeyathayaparan, S., Angunawala, P., Karnnanayake, E. H. and Jayasinghe, K. S. A. (1994) Effect of Momordica charantia on key hepatic enzymes. *Journal of Ethnopharmacology*, **44**, 93–97

ter Riet, G., Kleijnen, J. and Knipschild, P. (1990) Acupuncture and chronic pain: a criterion based meta-analysis. *Journal of Clinical Epidemiology*, **11**, 1191–1199

Tolge, C., Iyer, V. and McConnell, J. (1993) Phrenic nerve palsy accompanying chiropractic manipulation of the neck. *Southern Medical Journal*, **86**, 688–90

Tsukerman, I. M. (1970) A rare case of carcinoma of the skin arising after acupuncture. *Voprosy Onkologii*, **16**, 88

Vanhaelen, M., Vanhaelen, R., But, P. and Vanherweghem, J. L. (1994) Identification of aristolochic acid in Chinese herbs. *Lancet*, **i**, 174

Van Ulsen, J., Stolz, E. and Joost, T. (1988) Chromate dermatitis from a homoeopathic drug. *Contact Dermatitis*, **18**, 56–57

Vittecoq, D., Mettetal, J. F., Rouzioux, C., Bach, J. F. and Bouchon, J. P. (1989) Acute HIV infection after acupuncture treatments. *New England Journal of Medicine*, **320**, 250–51

Vlachos, P. and Kanitsakis, N. N. (1994) Fatal cardiac and renal failure due to *Ecbalium elaterium* (squirting cucumber). *Clinical Toxicology*, **32**, 737–738

Widler, P., Mathys, K., Brenneisen, R., Kalix, P. and Fisch, H. U. (1994) Pharmacodynamics and pharmacokinetics of khat: a controlled study. *Clinical Pharmacological Therapeutics*, **55**, 556–562

Wilkie, A. and Cordess, Ch. (1994) Ginseng – a root just like a carrot? *Journal of the Royal Society of Medicine*, **87**, 594–596

Woolf, G. M., Petrovic, L. M., Rojter, S. E., Wahwright, S., Villanil, F. G. and Katov, W. N. *et al.* (1994) Acute hepatitis associated with Chinese herbal product Jin Bu Huan. *Annals of Internal Medicine*, **121**, 729–735

Wright, R. S., Kupperman, J. L. and Liebhaber, M. I. (1991) Bilateral tension pneumothoraces after acupuncture. *Western Journal of Medicine*, **154**, 102–103

Yorston, D. and Foster, A. (1994) Traditional eye medicines and corneal ulceration in Tanzania. *Journal of Tropical Medicine and Hygiene*, **97**, 211–214

Chapter 9

Safety in complementary medicine

Wayne B. Jonas

Introduction

Complementary, alternative, and unconventional medical practices are increasing in popularity. In the USA, it has been estimated that at least one-third of the population uses these practices on a regular basis (Eisenberg *et al.*, 1993). In Europe the percentage is even higher, being from 40 to 70% in some cases (Fisher and Ward, 1994). The World Health Organization (WHO) estimates that 65–80% of the world's population depends upon traditional practices (mostly herbal preparations) for their health care management. As increasing and more extensive use of these practices spreads, their safety is also becoming of increasing concern (Ernst, 1995a). Toxic products can be used in a relatively safe manner, provided they are delivered in the context of good clinical training, a supporting medical infrastructure, and with close monitoring. Many of the practices used in complementary medicine involve self-care, or the delivery by non-medical practitioners – the adequacy of whose training is unknown, unmonitored, or inadequate (Ernst, 1995b). Thus, there is increasing potential for public harm with misuse of these practices. This situation calls for closer scrutiny of potential adverse effects from complementary medicine practices.

The relative nature of 'safety'

Safety is defined in Webster's dictionary as being, 'freedom from whatever exposes one to danger or from liability to cause danger or harm; safeness; hence the quality of making safe or secure or of giving confidence, justifying trust, insuring against harm or loss, etc'. It derives from the Sanskrit word *sarva*, which is akin to the word *salus*, meaning 'of sound condition, well-preserved, unharmed, whole'. It is thus intimately related with the concept of health and wholeness, or completeness, but refers more specifically to conditions which threaten such wholeness or health.

The medical application of safety, however, reveals it to be a relative term, as reflected by the fact that the United States' Food and Drug Administration, which is charged with ensuring safety of products and devices, has no specific definition of the term. Safe is relative to a number of factors, including:

1. The toxicity of the device or the product being used
2. The potential benefits incurred in using it
3. The context of use (such as self-care, under the care of a competently trained professional, with knowledge, skills and abilities for its proper use)
4. Appropriate monitoring, marketing, advertising, etc. so that its use is accessed properly
5. The values that underlie judgement of its proper use, such as the desired and expected outcomes and the often subjective judgements that go into determining whether its effects are adverse or beneficial.

To speak of safety, one must address the relative risk to benefit derived from engaging in such practices or administering products with therapeutic intent. This risk-benefit ratio, then becomes the index by which the relative safety is judged. For most issues of safety, only the direct assessment of the risk-benefit ratio can give us reliable information with which to make evidenced-based judgements about the safety of a practice.

The relative safety of 'natural'

A frequent reason that individuals give for turning to complementary and alternative medicine is that these products are often assumed to be safer than conventional medicine and drug therapy (O'Conner, 1995). Indeed, the term 'natural' medicine, as used frequently in Germany and elsewhere, is one of the attractive features of these practices for patients who may be frightened of the side effects from conventional therapies. They assume that therapies labelled 'natural' are inherently safer.

Some interventions and diagnostic practices that fall under the heading of complementary and alternative medicine do, on the surface, appear to be inherently safe. Examples include meditation, patient education, mind-body techniques such as visualization, psychic, or spiritual healing, and to a great extent, whole systems of practice such as homoeopathy and acupuncture. Other complementary therapies clearly present direct risks. Examples are herbal remedies, therapies such as intravenous hydrogen peroxide, high-dose megavitamin and mineral infusions, and procedures such as colonics, or high-velocity spinal manipulation. Yet, given the risk-benefit definition just described, can one assume that any therapy which, on the surface appears to be mostly harmless, is safe? Clearly the general answer to this must be no, but the type and degree of assurances, monitoring, and training required for their use must vary considerably. To ask the question, 'is complementary medicine safe?' is no more useful to ask than to ask, 'is medicine safe?' This can only be answered in the negative, as medicine itself is applied only when individuals are under duress from disease, illness, and suffering and, therefore, are willing to undergo manipulations, toxicity, and inconveniences not normally sought after or desired.

An example of the need to match appropriate criteria to specific complementary medicine therapies can be illustrated in the evaluation of homoeopathy. On the surface, it would appear that homoeopathy, which uses highly dilute and infrequently given substances is inherently safe. This may be largely true. Homoeopathic remedies often begin with highly toxic substances, but through a process of serial dilution end up having little or none of the toxic substance left in the final preparation. Homoeopathy as a system would appear to be inherently non-toxic and not require toxicity testing of every homoeopathic medicine. However, certain precautions apply. First, not all homoeopathic preparations, or preparations labelled 'homoeo-pathic' have extremely dilute substances. Some low potencies or homoeopathic preparations mixed with herbal products may have significant amounts of potentially dangerous substances (Kerr and Saryan, 1986).

Second, the general class of serial agitated dilutions or high 'potencies' in homoeopathy have never been adequately tested for their inherent safety. By this I mean they have never had direct preclinical toxicity tests done to determine if they truly do not have direct toxic effects. Is there any reason to be concerned about this? The homoeopathic literature is full of so-called 'provings' in which healthy volunteers are given, often highly dilute homoeopathic preparations and their subsequent symptoms meticulously recorded. This is akin to a phase I trial in drug testing and these 'provers' frequently report large numbers of symptoms, some of which can be serious. Proving symptoms are used to help guide the selection of homoeopathic remedies for therapeutic purposes. One would have to assume from this extensive proving literature that even high dilutions of homoeopathic preparations can potentially produce adverse effects. The provings themselves, unless done with sufficient numbers, over a long enough period of time, and in a double-blind, randomized fashion, cannot give information about the accuracy or extent of those effects. Recently, provings have incorporated these design mechanisms and may be able to provide some of these data. However, it would be unreasonable, from our current understanding of chemistry and pharmacology, to require that all remedies in high dilutions be demonstrated to have no toxicity. Rather, a more pragmatic approach would be to require both preclinical and phase I trials of high potencies (one might perhaps select five or six different medicines and five or six different 'doses') and observe if any objective or subjective and reliable effects are produced on an acute and chronic basis. There are reports in the old homoeopathic literature and literature from India of pathological changes in animals given high dilutions over long periods of time (Stearns, 1925; Chandrasekhar, Prasad and Rao, 1976).

Prayer might also be assumed to have no direct toxic effects and therefore, not require preclinical and phase I testing. Adverse effects from 'psychic' phenomena have been documented, however (Dossey, 1994). Whether or not one understands the mechanisms, (e.g. psychogenic, cultural, autonomic, or other) can we reasonably assume that such information has no inherent, acute, and serious adverse effects?

Therapies with known or suspected toxic effects (such as herbal preparations) may turn out to be inherently safer, given their relative benefits, than comparable conventional therapies. An example of this is the use of *Hypericum* (St John's wort) extract in the treatment of mild to moderate depression. The efficacy of this herb in the treatment of mild to moderate depression has been demonstrated in over a dozen clinical trials with very few and minor side effects. In direct comparison with conventional antidepressants, *Hypericum* has comparable efficacy yet fewer side effects (Linde *et al.*, 1995, in press). This illustrates that a therapy with higher potential direct toxic effects than homoeopathy or prayer may be inherently more desirable, i.e. 'safer' given the indications and comparative value to established conventional therapies, because of a reduced risk-benefit ratio. Thus, decisions about safety and relative safety may require evaluation using various criteria, both for a system as a whole, i.e. homoeopathy, prayer, herbalism, etc., and specific products within that system. Certain therapeutic systems, such as acupuncture and homoeopathy, may require only toxicity screening and appropriate training for their use as a whole system to be considered sufficiently safe for application. Specific product safety testing in this case for each indication would be unrealistic, hinder their delivery to the market, and generate numerous false-positive concerns or reports of adverse effects. Other interventions, such as herbalism, or megavitamin therapy would require both screening of the entire system of application for general safety characteristics and specific testing of standardized products for selected indications prior to marketing of these claims. An example of this approach is the World Health Organization's *Guidelines for Safe Acupuncture Treatment* (WHO, 1995), and the works ongoing now in several countries developing both safe and practical regulation of botanical products (Baker, 1990; Blackburn, 1993; Blumenthal and Klein, 1996) which include issues of quality manufacture techniques, standards for needle structure and size, materials, strength, sterilization procedures, packaging, and labelling, as well as standards of needling techniques to assure safety in depth, location and duration (Lao, 1994).

Components of safety

Adverse effects from complementary medical practices can be classified into three broad categories: direct, indirect, and definitional. Direct adverse effects are either short term in which they are labelled 'toxic effects' or long term in which they may be called 'side effects'. Indirect adverse effects are those events that occur because of the delivery practices of the therapy or diagnostic procedure in the context in which the practices apply, as opposed to direct physiological or physical impact from the intervention itself. Indirect effects can be classified into four categories: mislabelling, misrepresentation, misapplication, and misinformation. Finally, a full consideration of the safety of complementary medicine, especially the indirect effects, must consider the definitional aspects. Many systems of complementary medicine use completely different diagnostic categories, patient preferences, explanatory models, and outcome values than those commonly accepted in the West. Failure to provide clarity in these definitional and descriptional areas can lead to misunderstanding that can also produce adverse effects during application or attempted application of the practice.

Mislabelling

Mislabelling occurs when a product or device does not contain the items it is purported to contain or perform the actions it is stated to perform. In products such as herbal preparations, mislabelling may involve the application of a specific herbal name, and yet the product may not contain that herb. Confusion among the various ginseng products, for example, has lead to inaccurate claims for toxicity. Herbal products are sometimes labelled with a single herb, but actually contain products from a variety of plants (Awang, 1994).

Some homoeopathic products are labelled homoeopathic because they include highly dilute preparations combined with plant products or even pharmacological doses of conventional drugs. Likewise acupuncture needles may not be prepared with appropriate manufacturing and sterility standards and yet be labelled as sterile. Mislabelling can occur because good manufacturing processes and assessment procedures are not incorporated in the manufacture of the product, or they may occur deliberately to mislead the practitioner or patient in which case they are fraudulent. Direct and fraudulent mislabelling of products does occur, however, its frequency is unknown and probably represents a minority of products compared with those inadvertently mislabelled from inadequate manufacturing and standardization procedures.

While the extent of fraudulent mislabelling is largely unknown, a more significant subset of mislabelling is underlabelling. This occurs when potentially toxic ingredients and the concentrations of other potentially active ingredients are not on the label. For example, some traditional Chinese and ayurvedic herbal preparations may contain toxic doses of mercury, lead, arsenic and other heavy metals (Harper, 1994). In some cases these are either deliberately added or allowed to exist in such preparations and thought by the complementary medical system to be important for their therapeutic effects. These substances are clearly toxic, with especially long-term damaging effects if ingested by children, and do not appear on the label. Nor can the predictions about their concentration be estimated from the name of the plant product, or herbal mixture. The recent Food Supplement Labelling Act passed by the US Government has probably aggravated this problem in allowing some products that are most frequently used as therapeutic agents to be classified as foods. This results in less labelling of the content and appropriate usage of the products. Underlabelling can be just as serious as mislabelling.

Misrepresentation

Misrepresentation occurs from the incorporation of ineffective interventions or diagnostic procedures that are thought to be or are used as if effective. Even in relatively benign conditions, misrepresentation can result in adverse effects because of the risk of wasting time, money, the increased use of diagnostic techniques (including repeated history and physical examination), and the generation of false expectations about the outcome. In addition, misrepresentation of ineffective therapies can result in harm if truly effective therapies are not discovered or applied for the alleviation of the condition.

There are two key issues here. First is whether an intervention is needed at all. Many conditions have a benign, natural course or recover spontaneously and require no intervention. In these cases, any intervention carries potential risks. For example, close to 80% of individuals who visit a general practice and for whom a specific diagnosis is unobtainable will have their problem resolve or improve such that no therapy is subsequently needed (Thomas, 1974). In this case, any intervention with potential side effects, inconvenience, cost, or that produces anxiety or other psychological factors would be inappropriate. Thus prognostic need is an important part of defining misrepresentation. Failure to understand the prognosis of a condition in order to determine what may be a benign or serious illness can result in progression of an illness that might otherwise be arrested or interference with a condition that will heal itself. Increased self-care with natural medicines and the assumption of comprehensive medical care by practitioners without extensive experience and training in the management of serious disease, can lead to unfavourable, avoidable and, therefore, adverse outcomes. Examples of this have been published such as the attempted treatment of diabetes mellitus using ineffective herbal preparations (Ernst, 1995b). Other examples include the treatment of cancers in the early stages using biological or homoeopathic preparations and the reliance on prayer and mental healing while serious conditions progressed (Herbert and Kasdan, 1994). These cases may be rare but the true prevalence of such events from a public health perspective is unknown.

This aspect of misrepresentation can only occur if there is truly an effective conventional therapy for the condition. In many instances this is not the case as only about 20–50% of conventional practice is proven through appropriate clinical trials. For example, acupuncture or homoeopathic treatment may alleviate the pain and improve the function of osteoarthritis due to completely non-specific effects. Since the side effects of these therapies are less than those produced by anti-inflammatory drugs used in conventional medicine and since conventional treatment with non-steroidal anti-inflammatory drugs does not change the long-term prognosis of this disease, the use of these two alternative modalities in the treatment of arthritis could not be properly considered misrepresentation in this sense.

Ultimately determining the extent and accuracy of misrepresentation requires evidence from direct comparative trials of alternative medical practices. It is only through randomized comparative trials that optimal therapies (those with the least risk-benefit ratio) can be judged. Separate testing of alternative and conventional therapies against placebo or sham interventions with variable effects cannot be used to make determinations about relative effectiveness between therapies. Thus, the accuracy and true extent of misrepresentation must ultimately be determined by direct comparative trials.

Comparative trials
The number of direct comparative trials of complementary and alternative therapies compared with proven conventional therapies has increased. There are now a number of examples comparing acupuncture, homoeopathy and herbal preparations, as well as spinal manipulation and traditional Chinese medicine with and without incorporation of conventional medicine in randomized controlled trials. These trials, often, but not always, demonstrate similar efficacy with reduced adverse effects from complementary therapies.

Examples of such a direct comparison are the *Hypericum* versus imipramine trial (Vorbach, Hubner and Arnoldt, 1993), the comparison of classical homoeopathy versus salicylates in the treatment of rheumatoid arthritis (Gibson *et al.*, 1980), and the controlled trial comparing antacids, cimetidine, deglycyrrhizinated liquorice and gefarnate in the treatment of chronic duodenal ulceration (Cassir, 1985). In the latter trial, effects in the four groups were approximately the same but the deglycyrrhinizated liquorice showed considerably less side effects. Hammerschlag (1994) has summarized the direct comparative trials of acupuncture versus conventional medicine in a variety of conditions. In most trials where the efficacy (and indication of benefit) of conventional treatments is similar to acupuncture, side effects (an indication of risks) were usually less (Hammerschlag, 1994). More trials of this type are needed in complementary medicine.

Misapplication

Misapplication of effective therapies can also result in harm. This usually occurs because of inadequate training, in either knowledge skills or experience, resulting in suboptimal application of an intervention. Conventional medicine has well-established training, certification, licensing, and monitoring procedures to assure that the knowledge skills and qualifications of a practitioner are adequate. Even with these safeguards, misapplication occurs. If complementary and alternative practitioners engage in the entire scope of a medical practice then their knowledge skills and experience in these areas must be at least comparable to those involved in conventional primary care, or their practice should be specifically restricted and defined. Appropriate referral to and from medically qualified practitioners requires knowledge of which conditions are best managed and under what circumstances by those practitioners. As the number, type, and background of complementary practitioners increases and as the identification of more and more effective and ineffective complementary therapies occurs, a generalist gatekeeper and medical coordinator with knowledge of complementary and conventional medicine will be needed to prevent misapplication.

Misapplication can occur by conventional practitioners who may fail to refer to or apply effective complementary practices. The rise in schools of acupuncture for medically qualified doctors results in considerably less training and experience in acupuncture than that considered adequate in countries where extensive use and training of traditional acupuncturists has occurred for centuries. The WHO is attempting to address these problems by creating categories of acupuncturists with various training standards and scopes of practice. Thus minimum hours and standards for the training of qualified medical doctors in acupuncture are defined, as well as minimal training and experience in anatomy, physiology, pathophysiology, prognosis, and scope of practice for acupuncturists in Western diagnosis and medicine. Without such standards for all those who may engage in, refer to, or recommend complementary practices, misapplication is likely to continue unchecked. An example of how confusing these standards are in the USA can be seen in the acupuncture training, licensing, and accrediting regulations. There are at least three certifying bodies in acupuncture and Oriental medicine, each having different requirements for certification and scopes of practice. States seeking to provide appropriate laws for licensing and regulating acupuncturists, may use criteria from different organizations or from none of these organizations in their certification process. A similar situation exists with homoeopathic practitioners, having various certification, licensing and training requirements for doctors, nurses, dentists and even lay practitioners. Likewise, competition between multiple organizations for naturopathic training, licensing, and certification exists. These various organizations and practices are recognized inconsistently by different states. Whereas all 50 states recognize, license, and regulate chiropractors, only about 24 states have statutory regulations dealing with acupuncture, 12 with naturopathy, and four dealing with homoeopathy, one of which dates back to 1906. The situation in the UK is even more chaotic, where the practice of complementary medicine does not require certification or licensing at all.

Misinformed application

Finally, harm can occur because of misinformed application by skilled practitioners. This occurs mostly because of incorrect, inaccurate, or inappropriate diagnosis and patient classification, resulting in the application of effective therapies, but for the incorrect outcome, or because of failure to detect outcomes that can be corrected. Misinformed application because of inappropriate or inadequate diagnosis is different from misapplication of effective therapies because they are suboptimal. This has to do with clinical disagreement and diagnostic accuracy, or failure to detect and apply the therapy to the main cause of a condition, rather than to a minor contributing factor of the condition. There are many examples of complementary and alternative therapies that appear to create their own diagnosis for which their therapy is then applied. An example of this is iridology, which makes claims to diagnose specific conditions from patterns in the eye. Iridologists claim to be able to detect signs of disease early by looking at the eye and therefore, treatment can result in preventing the development of the full pathological condition. This results in unnecessary treatments or treatments that have not been proven to prevent that particular condition (Knipschild, 1988). Many other similar diagnostic methods are available, that in principle set up situations for the same risk. Electroacupuncture according to Voll for example, claims to be able to detect functional changes in acupuncture meridians and subsequently the corresponding organ locations which then become an 'electromagnetic' diagnosis of an existing or impending disease. These diseases created by the electroacupuncture instrument are then 'treated' using a variety of means. Without subsequent proof that such a diagnosis would indeed develop, these treatments claim to be 'preventive' and patients may go through multiple electroacupuncture measurements and 'treatments'. This causes harm by creating anxiety, excessive and unnecessary testing, treatments and expenditures of time and energy, all of which have unknown benefit. Similar complementary and alternative medical diagnostic systems including combinations of endocrinological and blood measurements from normal serum, radiathesia, intuitive diagnosis, auricular diagnosis, pleomorphism, etc., which all carry the same risk of misinformed application and misdiagnosis.

Orthodox medicine has its share of similar questionable screening and diagnostic methods, including tests such as prostate specific antigen, occult stool blood tests, fetal monitoring in normal pregnancies, and possibly other types of screening. In many of these tests, their reliability and correlation with significant outcomes is questionable, yet their application leads to interventions, all of which carry risks. Indeed, the tendency of conventional medicine to pay excessive attention to the medically 'correct' (objective, proven, most common, verifiable, most highly technical, etc.) outcomes at the expense of time spent attending to subjective, quality of life, and individually valued outcomes that are of importance to patients is probably a major reason why people turn to complementary and alternative practitioners (O'Conner, 1995). These are the definitional and value issues that, if not addressed, can also lead to adverse effects from treatment.

Definitional issues

The third domain that must be considered in assessing the safety of complementary practices are definitional issues. These revolve around the so-called 'model validity' of such practices. Many complementary practices are derived from the medical systems of non-western cultures, or carry basic epistemological assumptions about the nature of man and reality that are quite different from conventional science and medicine. These areas must be considered in order to prevent misunderstanding that may arise around different values underlying these practices. Model validity can impact safety judgments in five areas:

1. Definitions of the constituents or activity of a product.
2. Diagnostic taxonomy and patient classifications.
3. Type of outcomes valued by the complementary medical system.
4. The personal value placed by individuals on outcomes.
5. The explanatory model that drives the foregoing as well as what is considered relevant for hypothesis testing in research.

Product constituents

The safety of various products may revolve around how the medical system classifies what are important elements in those products, what constitutes purity, or the 'active ingredient'. Western biomedicine focuses almost exclusively on the chemical composition of products with the idea of identifying the molecular components that may lead to benefit or harm. Other complementary practices, however, may not consider the chemical component in determining the composition of their products. Traditional Chinese medicine, for example, involves a number of ancient formulae involving multiple plant combinations. Each plant complex is put together in order to provide a certain 'Qi' balance or have a 'Qi' effect in specific meridian systems in the body. Chemical composition is not a consideration. Likewise, ayurvedic medicine will combine certain massage techniques, sounds, and smells to balance out certain traditional 'qualities' or 'doshes' present in herbal and drug products. These 'qualities' are used without regard for the chemical constituents of the plant. Differing definitions of what is considered important in a product may conflict. This is especially apparent in the area of toxicity when heavy metal contamination is discovered in some of these preparations. These are considered toxic from the western chemical perspective but from the traditional medical perspective may be considered important for the therapeutic Qi or quality balancing effect.

Diagnostic taxonomy

Diagnostic taxonomy and patient classification comprise another area where definitional components can impact on safety. Western medicine has a set of disease classifications (mostly developed over the last 200 years), with associated prognosis and aetiologies that explain their signs and symptoms. These taxonomies are not considered uniform populations from the traditional perspective. A single western diagnosis, for example, low back pain or arthritis, when looked at from the traditional Chinese medicine perspective, may consist of 10 or 12 completely different diagnostic types, each requiring different treatment. Likewise, homoeopathy uses specific 'remedy pictures' as the basis for determining effective therapy. Different symptom pictures in patients with the same conventional biomedical diagnosis will receive different remedies and have different prognoses. Failure to consider a system's taxonomy can result in inappropriate research, claims of effectiveness or lack of effectiveness, and contribute to misapplication and misinformation. For example, Shipley and colleagues selected the homoeopathic remedy *Rhus toxicum*, considered to be the most effective for osteoarthritis patients, and applied it in a double-blind, placebo-controlled manner (Shipley *et al.*, 1983). The remedy demonstrated no effect. Homoeopathic practitioners, however, do not treat osteoarthritis with a single remedy, but only a subtype of arthritis with symptoms consistent with that remedy. Fisher subsequently evaluated patients with the western diagnosis of fibromyalgia, then selected out of this a subset whose symptoms fitted those for the same homoeopathic remedy *Rhus toxicum*. The remedy was then tested on this subset of patients in a randomized, double-blind, placebo-controlled fashion and found to be effective (Fisher *et al.*, 1989). From the homoeopathic perspective the Shipley trial and subsequent recommendation was an example of misinformed application leading to erroneous and therefore harmful conclusions.

Insisting on obtaining a western diagnosis because there is more objective information about aetiology and prognosis for this system may not provide optimal safety and effectiveness. For example, it is not unusual for a western diagnosis to provide details about prognosis and pathophysiology without providing adequate treatment for the alleviation of that condition. This is especially true in many chronic diseases. For example, the diagnosis of chronic pain syndrome may involve great description and detail of the contributing factors to its aetiology. This may result in the application of numerous types of psychotherapeutic, physical and pharmacological therapies, each with their subsequent direct and indirect risks. This diagnostic classification, however, often reaches an impasse, providing no further therapeutic benefit, but simply increased risks from more intense and detailed therapies. Assessment of the patient from an ayurvedic or a traditional Chinese perspective, however, may provide an alternative conceptualization of the patient, allowing for similar outcomes with less intervention and therefore risks. A similar situation arises in the treatment of advanced solid tumours. Conventional diagnostic theory and pathophysiology involves a paradigm in which the tumour cells are the focus of destructive therapy. This focus on 'killing' the pathological diagnosis, eventually results in an impasse without further advancement or discovery of productive therapies. An alternative diagnostic classification of advanced cancer conditions that incorporate biological and psychological modifiers of the cancer condition, may result in alternative approaches to these conditions, more relevant than the clinical and aetiogical taxonomy.

Outcome substitution
The third definitional issue involves the outcome values in complementary and alternative medicine. Patients using various complementary approaches may value different outcomes than that of western biomedicine. Western biomedicine focuses on cure, which is the elimination of the pathognomonic or diagnostic condition. Other approaches such as nursing, may emphasize care, which involves helping patients cope with suffering and attending to the personal dimensions of the chronic condition. Some complementary and alternative practices emphasize the importance of acceptance and use of the disease as a guide to personal improvement. Still others may classify some signs and symptoms as important signals indicating recovery rather than illness. In homoeopathy, for example, we have the frequent statement that to see an aggravation of symptoms after a drug is given (which in conventional medicine would be considered a side effect) is a good sign that predicts comprehensive improvement in the future. Finally, some complementary systems have as their main outcome, what I call enlightenment, that is that the goal of the condition and therapy are both for a change in perception of life. The goal of 'therapy' is discovering meaning in the suffering and thereby

growing in wisdom. Many mind-body, psychic, and spiritualist healing based systems incorporate this as one of their primary outcomes. Different outcome variables are often not explicit in these systems, leading to misunderstanding and inappropriate application of the therapy.

Patient values and autonomy

An extension of the problem with misunderstanding related to the outcome goals of some complementary practices involves understanding the personal value system of the patient. Research, by necessity, groups patients according to certain outcomes and assesses the impact of specific interventions on those outcomes. Individual patients within that group, however, may value alternative outcomes than those which are under study. If these personal outcome values are not considered, then the intervention, studied for its effect on single or limited outcomes, risks misapplication because of misunderstanding. This is personal outcome substitution in which the diagnostic category does not fit the patient preference in therapy. For example, a patient with arthritis may receive conventional treatment aimed at improving pain and reducing inflammation, whereas the individual patient may desire increased function and regard pain and inflammation as less important or a secondary goal. Alternatively, a third patient may be more concerned with prolonged suffering, general well-being, long-term outcomes, or the possibility of death and disability from the diagnosis. They may find intervention directed at pain, inflammation, or function to be secondary to obtaining the knowledge and skills for coping with their illness. Failure to consider personal preferences, explanations, and values, both from the complementary model and the patient's perspective, can result in misunderstanding and thus misapplication of even effective therapy by well-trained practitioners.

The explanatory model

Understanding the explanatory model of the culture in which the therapy is delivered can also impact on judgement about indirect adverse effects. Kleinman demonstrated, for example, that traditional healers frequently and almost inevitably heal. Their patients are usually satisfied claiming the therapies are effective without important side effects, when by western criteria the therapies are not considered effective. Without detailed explanation of such values, defining what is an adverse or beneficial effect may become problematic for assessing risk-benefit ratios (Kleinman, 1981).

Tools for safety assessment in complementary medicine

Clinical accuracy

Modern science has derived a number of methods for attempting to assess safety of conventional medical practices. Despite this safety net, it is not infrequent to find significant risks being uncovered after years of use (ultraviolet light treatments, calcium channel blockers, prostate cancer surgery, etc.). For practical purposes, the methods needed to detect adverse events are the same both for the indirect and the long-term direct effects. Direct, short-term toxicological effects are much easier (depending upon severity) but, in some cases, can be exaggerated or underdetected without proper investigative design. First, it should be kept in mind that there is often wide clinical disagreement about whether a particular adverse effect was due to a therapy. Even pharmacologists, for example, disagreed 36% of the time as to whether or not a particular adverse effect was due to a drug. The rate of disagreement goes up the more the serious the attribution, with a 50% disagreement on whether an admission to the hospital was due to an adverse drug reaction and a 71% disagreement that a death was due to an adverse drug reaction (Koch-Weser, Sellers and Zachest, 1977).

Methods of measurement

Second, current methods of surveying for adverse effects, even in clinical trials, by using broad checklists, patient interviews or questionnaires, is unlikely to yield relevant associations. For example, using symptom checklists to monitor symptoms attributable to adverse drug reactions resulted in 81% of individuals checking yes, with a mean of two symptoms per individual, and 7% reporting six or more symptoms (Reidenberg and Lowenthal, 1968). Most symptoms collected in this way will be false positive. The true rate of adverse events, even in extensively used therapies, may not be detected without rigorously designed, hypothesis-driven, prospective trials with groups randomized to the intervention and a control group.

Rare events and public health impact

Since adverse events occur rarely for many complementary medical practices (Awang, 1994; Ernst, 1994; Perharic et al., 1994; Ernst, 1995a,c; WHO, 1995), relatively large numbers (i.e. 3 × 1000 over the inverse ratio of events) and special designs are needed to be 95% confident that even one adverse event would be detected. Adverse drug reporting can significantly underestimate these effects as only

5–10% of such events are ever reported. On the other hand, non-random cohort or case-control evaluations of adverse events often over-inflate estimates of events with odds ratios of even two or three subsequently being found to be false (La Haba *et al.*, 1971). Because of their widespread use complementary and alternative interventions may have significant public health implications. Accurately assessing the adverse effects of a single complementary medicine therapy would require post-marketing surveillance of upwards of 3000 individuals. In addition, the rate of rare idiosyncratic and allergic reactions needs similar, large-scale post-marketing assessment (De Smet, 1995).

Types of evidence in adverse effects assessment

There are various types of evidence often used for reporting on safety in medicine, each with their usefulness and limitations. First, pre-clinical evidence can often give indications of areas where there is potential toxicity and guide hypothesis testing and mechanism studies. Such information may identify compounds of potentially high risks in humans, but cannot be automatically inferred to be harmful in the context of their clinical use. For example, phenobarbital increases the rate of hepatacellular carcinoma in rats, but when prepared as an homoeopathic dilution can result in decreased rates of such cancers (De Gerlache and Lans, 1991).

Historical evidence is often used to indicate that natural products are self-evidently safe. Historical evidence is useful for giving general indications about acute toxicity. However, given the different morbidity and mortality curves and uses of such products in the modern age, such evidence cannot be used to indicate potential chronic effects or indirect risks. Therefore, this type of evidence is not useful for making firm conclusions about the value of these products in practice (Huxtable, 1994).

Case reports in the literature are the most frequent method of illustrating and emphasizing potential toxicity from complementary treatments. Such reports on adverse effects have the same limitations that anecdotal reports of beneficial effects have from the proponents of such practices. These reports allow for more detailed descriptions of possible adverse associations, but cannot be used to make any indications about frequency or possible attribution of those effects from the therapy. These reports can only tell us that adverse events can occur, not that they must occur or even did occur, nor how frequently and, as in anecdotal reports about benefit, they are likely to lead to an over-interpretation of the significance of such events. Lists of such anecdotal reports have been collected in the literature for a number of practices (especially herbal practices, acupuncture, megavitamin therapy) (Peacher, 1975; Herbert and Kasdan, 1994). Most authors agree that many of the more established complementary, alternative, and traditional medical interventions do not produce many serious adverse reactions when used in the traditional and/or indicated manner. Post-marketing surveillance can give information about the prevalence and incidence, and some frequency and association data. As discussed previously, however, these often require large numbers (1000 plus) to identify with any confidence the reliability of adverse events rates. Such approaches risk inflating those events, however, because specifically searching for events among a population can lead to search intensity bias, even in case-controlled studies (Reidenberg and Lowenthal, 1968). These studies must be conducted using objective outcome measures in a way that provides equal opportunity for finding and extracting information from exposed and unexposed groups. Failure to use blind evaluations can lead to diagnostic suspicion bias which also can inflate and exaggerate the rate of these events (Sackett et al., 1993).

Adverse effect reporting registries, such as MedWatch used by the FDA in the USA, can provide an indication of the popularity or rising use of new therapies, or about changes in opinions in the value of new therapies in practice. On occasion, they can be used to identify new unexpected problems, such as sudden delayed acute or chronic reactions from treatment exposures. These registries, however, are notoriously subject to falsification and without rigorous verification methods built in cannot be relied on for accuracy or prevalence data.

Information on adverse reactions also often comes from data collected at poison control centres. These data are valuable for the likelihood of adverse reactions that occur mostly through misuse and abuse of therapies (self-medication, suicide, fraudulent practices, accidents, etc.) (Perharic et al., 1994). These sources of data cannot provide information about safety under conditions of appropriate therapeutic use, nor is the accuracy of such information high, given the high rates of disagreement about true adverse drug effects indicated previously.

Phase I and phase II controlled trials are the only rigorous designs that can begin to indicate attributional effects. As indicated previously, however, the usual methods of collection of adverse effects using open-ended checklists increases the risk of missing the real effects secondary to multiple outcome assessments. In addition, the small size of these trials and their usual short-term duration reduce the chance of detecting small numbers of significant effects or those that may be delayed.

Phase III true efficacy trials allow us to make conclusions about attribution and are likely to be accurate if properly conducted.

However, as indicated above, unless the adverse effects themselves are not hypothesis generated, real adverse effects may be obscured by the high likelihood of obtaining positive associations. In addition, many complementary and alternative practices may find adequate sham controls problematic. For example, sham acupuncture usually shows increased effects over no acupuncture but less effects than 'real' acupuncture, indicating that both specific and non-specific effects occur (Hammerschlag, 1994). Likewise, delivery of sham acupuncture cannot be done blind in a way that allows a reasonable approximation of how the therapy is delivered in clinical practice. Such trials may necessitate a pragmatic orientation that can never positively identify adverse effects from the specific therapy. If such effects are low to begin with, identifying these effects unequivocally may be impractical and unnecessary. The most valuable type of evidence would be hypothesis-generated toxicity studies done in randomized placebo-controlled fashion (with randomized clinical trials). This has the highest likelihood of showing true accurate adverse effects; however, because of its complexity, it is rarely done. Even hypothesis-generated, randomized clinical trials for toxicity, however, will not illuminate outcome substitution bias, in which more easily measured or objective outcomes become the focus of the study, when less easily measured or subjective outcomes are the most relevant for the patients involved. This is the proverbial drunk looking for his lost car keys under the lamp where there is more light, though he lost them in the dark.

Finally, none of these types of evidence adequately addresses the issue of model validity and the complexities that arise in attempting to assess optimal therapy (treatment of choice). This information comes best from direct randomized comparative trials and trials that incorporate patient preferences and outcome measures pertinent to the complementary system under investigation. (Trials that have good individual and model fit.)

The safety of selected complementary practices by evidence type

Ernst and others have catalogued a number of case reports of adverse effects published in the literature from cervical manipulation, acupuncture, herbals, and homoeopathy (Ernst, 1994, 1995a,c). Perharic et al. (1994) have surveyed the toxicological problems resulting from traditional remedies and food supplements reported to a poison control centre. Of the 5536 contacts, 657 (12%) had symptoms indicative of adverse effects from the ingestion. Most of

Table 9.1 Poison control centres – reports relating to traditional remedy and food supplement ingestion

Item	Number	Percentage
Total reports	5536	100
Symptoms	657	12
Probable link to ingestion	42	< 1
Vitamins	342/4019	8
Food supplements	17/141	12
Herbal products	245/968	25

From Perharic *et al.* (1994)

these were children under 5 years who had ingested vitamins in overdose. Forty-two of these had a probability of being linked to the ingestion and two a high probability. The rates of adverse effects were calculated and for vitamins were 342 in 4019 (8%), for food supplements 17 in 141 (12%), and for herbal products 245 in 968 (25%) (Table 9.1).

Randomized controlled trials of adverse effects in alternative and complementary medicine published in the conventional peer-reviewed literature

Adverse effects reported in randomized controlled trials of alternative and complementary medicine as published in the conventional peer-reviewed literature would be the best type of evidence for identifying the true rate of hypothesis-driven, attributable, adverse effects from the proper use of such interventions under normal conditions. This is because it is unlikely that inflated effects would be found from blinded trials using randomized assignment to therapy, that were specifically reporting on adverse effects and published in non-advocacy journals. Though the number of such studies may be small, such an approach would provide the most accurate assessment of direct risks attributable to complementary medicine under the conditions of appropriate experimental use. In order to access this information, we examined all the citations from the National Library of Medicine (MEDLARS System) that dealt with alternative and complementary medicine, from blinded, double-blind, randomized control trials that specifically looked for and reported on adverse effects. Studies that involved extracted or purified plant toxins (e.g. podophyllotoxin) that were being used in combination with or as chemotherapeutic agents for cancer or were in common use in conventional medicine such as transcutaneous electrical nerve stimulation therapy, direct electrical muscle stimulation, conventional chemotherapeutic agents (vincristine), etc. were excluded from the study.

One hundred and twenty-one studies were found by combining alternative medicine, randomized controlled trials, double blind, and adverse effects. Of these, 27 were found to meet the inclusion criteria and were evaluated for the type of therapy, the duration of the trial, diagnosis and indication, the number in the trial, and the rate of adverse effects as compared with the control group (either conventional therapy or placebo). For therapies compared with conventional therapies we assessed whether the rate of adverse effects was lower, higher or equal and for the placebo trials whether the therapeutic efficacy of the trial was positive. Twenty-two of the studies involved plant or herbal preparations, two used megadose vitamins, two traditional Chinese medicine, and one electromagnetic pulsed fields. Mean duration of the trials was 10.3 weeks (range of 1 to 52 weeks, standard deviation 11.4 weeks). The type of condition ranged from cholesterol reduction and hayfever to nephrotic syndrome and advanced cancer. The average number of patients enrolled in the trial was 89 with a range of 15 to 263 and a standard deviation of 73.1 (Table 9.2).

The total number of adverse effects in those studies that reported on the patient numbers was 17 out of 565 patients (3%). Nine studies compared the complementary with the conventional therapy in a direct randomized fashion. Of these, six reported decreased side effects from a complementary therapy. All six of these reported that

Table 9.2 The rate of adverse effects

- Randomized controlled trials of alternative medicine
- Double blind
- Mcdline tagged 'Adverse effects'
- Excluded
  Psychotherapy, TENS, podophyllotoxin
  Muscle stimulation, chemotherapy
- 121 found; 27 included
- 27 studies; 22 plants, 2 vitamins, 2 traditional Chinese medicine, 1 electromagnetic pulsed fields
- Mean trial duration 10.3 weeks (s.d.11.4)
- Mean $n = 89$ (s.d.73.1)
- Total adverse effects = 17/565 or 3%
- 9 studies direct comparison of complementary and conventional medicine
  6 decreased adverse effects of complementary medicine
  1 increased adverse effect of complementary medicine
  2 no difference

the complementary therapy was equally efficacious as the conventional therapy for the condition. Only one study reported increased side effects from a complementary therapy and this involved one additional patient with an adverse effect out of 33 treated with the herb *Serenoa repens* for benign prostatic hypertrophy. The two remaining direct, comparative trials reported equal rates of adverse effects in both complementary and conventional therapy. Two studies carried out in developing countries using megadoses of vitamin A in healthy children are not included in these numbers. Both of these very large trials reported an increased rate of short-term (within 24 hours) vomiting, diarrhoea, colds, rhinitis, and coughs among those receiving the megadose of vitamin A instead of placebo. Odds ratios were extremely small, in the range of 1.02 to 1.18.

Assessing the use of complementary medical therapies under conditions which minimize indirect adverse effects and maximize an accurate estimate of attribution indicates an adverse effect rate of approximately 3%. The majority of studies that reported equal efficacy when directly comparing a complementary (usually herbal) intervention with a conventional drug therapy reported less side effects (six of nine) or equal side effects (two of nine). Only one of nine studies in this category reported a slightly increased rate (one out of 33 patients) over the conventional therapy. It is important to note that the duration of these studies was short, mean 10.3 weeks, and the total numbers in each group small (mean $n = 45$ per arm).

Conclusion

It appears that complementary medicine must deal seriously with the issue of safety and establish systems for addressing the direct, indirect and definitional issues that impact on the risk-benefit ratio of these practices. Purity and standardization of both the products and the training (competence) in these practices is primary. Without assurance of a good product and a well-trained practitioner to deliver the therapy, the risk-benefit ratio will be higher than necessary. The prevalence of adverse effects in homoeopathy, acupuncture, manipulation, herbal products, and mind-body therapies appears to be low, probably lower than comparable therapies in conventional medicine. These therapies are also at low risk for acute toxicity if used short term in the traditional manner or in controlled trials.

Important exceptions to this general rule exist, however. Especially of concern is possible heavy metal contamination of traditional herbal products. Almost no good data exist on the potential long-term adverse effects that might occur from chronic use of these practices.

In addition to the problems of competency, it appears that many alternative diagnostic systems have been inadequately tested and pose a real risk of exposing individuals to unnecessary anxiety, assessments, interventions, and costs. Misuse and poisonings do occur with symptomatic rates of approximately 12%. True attributable adverse effect rates appear to be in the range of 3%, especially for herbal and vitamin products and probably less for practices such as homoeopathy, acupuncture and mind/body therapies. Safety testing is needed, using appropriate hypothesis-generated, prospective, randomized methods with blind evaluators. It must include both preclinical and clinical trials firstly for certain complementary systems as a whole, such as homoeopathy, acupuncture, and various mind-body approaches; and also for specific products that have indications in specific conditions, such as herbal medications, megadose vitamins and minerals, and other biological products.

Finally, methods for reporting toxicity and adverse effects need improvement. Current systems used in conventional medicine must be applied with a specific understanding of their usefulness and limitations in providing accurate information about safety. Information from poison control centres, adverse effect reporting hotlines, post-marketing surveillance studies, preclinical research, and phase I and II trials all have different yet important limitations for determining the true attributable incidence and severity of adverse effects from complementary medical practices. Safety, as efficacy, must be evaluated under the conditions of proper use in order for improper use and misuse to be identified. Ultimately, only direct randomized comparative trials can give us the relative risk-benefit ratios needed for judging optimal therapy and the extent of misapplication. In the meantime, assessing the risks of misuse, educating the public about proper use, indications (versus claims) and precautions, and assuring competency of the practitioners who use and refer for complementary and alternative medicine is the best way to assure the safety and benefit of these practices.

References

Awang, D. D. C. (1996) *The Information Base for Safety Assessment of Botanicals.* OAM/FDA Sponsored Symposium on Botanicals: A Role in US Health Care. Washington, DC (in press)

Baker, C. C. (1990) *Report of the South Australian Working Party on Natural and Nutritional Substances.* South Australian Health Commission

Blackburn, J. L. C. (1993) *Second Report of the Expert Advisory Committee on Herbs and Botanical Preparations to the Health Protection Branch.* Health Canada, Ministry of Health, Canada

Blumenthal, M. and Klein, S. T. (eds.) (1996) *Therapeutic Monographs on Medicinal Plants for Human Use by Commission E Special Expert Committee of the German Federal Health Agency.* Austin: American Botanicals Council

Cassir, Z. A. (1985) Endoscopic control trial of four regimes in the treatment of chronic duodenal ulceration. *Irish Medical Journal*, **78**, 153–165

Chandrasekhar, K., Prasad, S. and Rao, C. V. (1976) Effect of pulsatilla nigra, a homoeopathic drug, on the uteri and estrus cycles in albino rats. *Journal of Research of Indian Medical Homeopathy*, **11**, 48–55

De Gerlache, J. and Lans M. (1991) Modulation of experimental rat liver carcinogenesis by ultra low doses of the carcinogens. *Ultra Low Doses*, edited by C. Doutremepuich. Washington, DC: Taylor & Francis. pp. 17–27

De Smet, P. A. G. M. (1995) Health risks of herbal remedies. *Drug Safety*, **13**, 233–45

Dossey, L. (1994) Healing and the mind: is there a dark side? *Journal of Scientific Exploration*, **8**, 73–90

Eisenberg, D. M., Kessler, R. C., Foster, C., Norlock, F. E., Collins, D. R. and Delbano, T. L. (1993) Unconventional medicine in the United States: prevalence, costs, and patterns of use. *New England Journal of Medicine*, **328**, 246–252

Ernst, E. (1994) Cervical manipulation: Is it really safe? *International Journal of Risk and Safety in Medicine*, **6**, 145–149

Ernst, E. (1995a) Bitter pills of nature: safety issues in complementary medicine. *Pain*, **60**, 237–238

Ernst, E. (1995b) Competence in complementary medicine. *Complementary Therapies in Medicine*, **3**, 6–8

Ernst, E. (1995c) The risks of acupuncture. *International Journal of Risk and Safety in Medicine*, **6**, 179–186

Fisher, P., Greenwood, A., Huskisson, E. C., Turner, P. and Belon, P. (1989) Effect of homoeopathic treatment on fibrositis (primary fibromyalgia). *British Medical Journal*, **299**, 365–366

Fisher, P. and Ward, A. (1994) Complementary medicine in Europe. *British Medical Journal*, **309**, 107–111

Gibson, R. G., Gibson, S., MacNeill, A. D. and Watson, B. W. (1980) Homoeopathic therapy in rheumatoid arthritis: evaluation by double-blind clinical trial. *British Journal of Clinical Pharmacology*, **9**, 453–459

Hammerschlag, R. (1994) *Survey of comparative outcomes research: clinical trials comparing acupuncture to standard medical treatment.* Proceedings of the Society for Acupuncture Research. Washington, DC: SAR

Harper, P. (1994) Traditional Chinese medicine for eczema. *British Medical Journal*, **308**, 489–490

Herbert, V. and Kasdan, T. S. (1994) Misleading nutrition claims and their gurus. *Nutrition Today*, **29**, 28–35

Huxtable, R. J. (1996) *Safety of botanicals: Historical perspective.* OAM/FDA Sponsored Symposium on Botanicals: A Role in US Health Care. Washington, DC: American Botanical Council monograph (in press)

Kerr, H. D. and Saryan, L. A. (1986) Arsenic content of homoeopathic medicines. *Clinical Toxicology*, **24**, 451–459

Kleinman, A. (1981) *Patients and Healers in the Context of Culture.* Berkeley, CA: University of California Press

Knipschild, P. (1988) Looking for gall bladder disease in the patient's iris. *British Medical Journal*, **287**, 1578–1581

Koch-Weser, J., Sellers, E. M. and Zachest, R. (1977) The ambiguity of adverse drug reactions. *European Journal of Clinical Pharmacology*, **11**, 75

La Haba, A., Curet, J., Pelegria, A. and Bangdiwala, I. (1971) Thrombophlebitis among oral and non-oral contraceptive users. *Obstetrics and Gynecology*, **38**, 259

Lao, L. (1996) *Safety Issues in Acupuncture*. OAM/FDA Sponsored Symposium on Acupuncture, Washington, DC: American Botanical Council Monograph (in press)

O'Conner, B. B. (1995) *Healing Traditions*. Philadelphia: University of Pennsylvania Press

Peacher, W. C. (1975) Adverse reactions, contraindications and complications of acupuncture and moxibustion. *American Journal of Chinese Medicine*, **3**, 35–46

Perharic, L., Shaw, D., Colbridge, M., House, I., Leon, C. and Murray, V. (1994) Toxicological problems resulting from exposure to traditional remedies and food supplements. *Drug Safety*, **11**, 264–294

Reidenberg, M. M. and Lowenthal, D. T. (1968) Adverse drug reactions. *New England Journal of Medicine*, **279**, 678

Sackett, D. L., Haynes, R. B., Guyatt, G. H. and Tugwell, P. (eds.) (1993) Deciding whether your treatment has done harm. In: *Clinical Epidemiology: A Basic Science for Clinical Medicine*. Boston: Little, Brown & Co

Shipley, M., Berry, H., Broster, G., Jenkins, M., Clover, A. and Williams, I. (1983) Controlled trial of homoeopathic treatment of osteoarthritis. *Lancet*, **i**, 97–98

Stearns, G. (1925) Completion of the experiment with high dilutions of natrum muriaticum given to guinea pigs. *Journal of the American Institute of Homeopathy*, **18**, 790–792

Thomas, K. B. (1974) Temporarily dependent patients in general practice. *British Medical Journal*, **1**, 625–626

Vorbach, E. U., Hubner, W. D. and Arnoldt, K. H. (1993) Wirksamkeit und Vertäglichkeit des Hypericum-Extraked LI 160 im Vergleich mit imipramin. *Nervenheilkunde*, **12**, 290–296

WHO. (1995) *Guidelines for Safe Acupuncture Treatment*. Geneva: World Health Organization

Chapter 10

The growth of complementary therapy: a consumer-led boom

David P. S. Dickinson*

Introduction

There is a boom in complementary medicine, and it is a boom that is consumer-led. More and more people are using complementary therapies: one in four during the last 12 months in a recent *Which?* survey (*Which?*, 1995), as against one in seven in 1986 (*Which?*, 1986). Many people are using these therapies as an adjunct to orthodox treatment, or for long-term problems that orthodox medicine has failed to fix. They are using them as a supplement to orthodox medicine, not as a substitute for it. People will often visit a complementary therapist with, say, a bad back for which the doctor can offer no further help. As a result, perhaps, general practitioners and other orthodox health professionals are taking more interest than ever before, in offering patients therapy themselves, or referring them to reliable practitioners.

For the moment, however, the greatest part of the money being paid for complementary therapies is overwhelmingly from private consultations. Private fees have been estimated to outsize NHS-paid fees by a factor of between 50 and 100:1 (White, personal communication). Our own survey showed just 6% of respondents having complementary treatment on the NHS (*Which?*, 1995). The growth of complementary care is privately funded, i.e., funded by consumers. It is logical that the relationship between therapist and patient needs to become more of a consumer transaction if complementary care is to continue to grow. A consumerist attitude – broadly, the provision of a safe and reliable service, with lots of information and a pro-active approach to complaints and feedback – is running through the National Health Service. Wherever complementary medicine is provided, the same attitudes need to take shape.

Consumerism in the relationship between patient and complementary therapist may take several forms.

Handling complaints. Work in both orthodox and complementary

*With special thanks to Gerry Cooney

therapy sectors shows that patients have in the past been unwilling to complain about substandard or dubious care (*Health Which?*, 1995). In private care, whether orthodox or complementary, they have often found themselves unable to complain if they needed to. Dissatisfied customers of complementary medicine still constitute a small minority: fewer it appears than those wishing to complain about orthodox medicine. But this may not last. It is clear that more people are complaining about orthodox medicine, and 1996 sees a new NHS system designed specifically to handle and even solicit complaints. Complaints will go up as a result of this system. This does not necessarily mean that NHS care is getting worse, but in a more consumerist atmosphere, more people are willing to complain and make their voices heard.

As complementary therapy matures in the UK it is likely to follow a similar pattern. As a part of the information revolution, its patients will become more knowledgeable about what to expect from treatment, and aware of good or bad practice. They will be more confident of their rights, more consumerist, and more willing to complain. At that point, complementary therapies and the bodies that represent them will (like hospitals or even business enterprises) start to be judged by how well they handle complaints, and how well they react to the small minority of people who have cause for complaint.

High expectations, good information. If disillusion plays a part in pushing many people towards complementary therapy, some users today harbour illusions once they are using it. There seems to be a general belief in the safety of treatments, usually expressed as a perception that they are more benign or natural than orthodox treatments, or less prone to side effects than drug-based orthodoxy. There is little or no information getting through to most people about which therapies are most appropriate for which conditions, or what outcomes can be expected. Consumers also want to know what treatment will cost. Misinformation benefits nobody. Therapists should be clear about their own and their colleagues' shortcomings (if any), about the risks inherent in any form of therapy, and what it can and cannot do. They should be openly sharing this information with their customers – just as we now demand clear information and openness from other health professionals. If information does not come from professional sources, it will be less reliable as it begins to be pumped down the line by any Tom, Dick or Harriet with a modem.

Standards and trust. It will come as a shock to patients, used to the compulsory registration of professionals within the NHS, that complementary practitioners need not have any academic or vocational qualifications, do not need to carry insurance nor belong to any registering body before they practise. People may also feel a false sense of security about individual therapists, preferring to trust their instinct to the chore of checking a register. There is compelling evidence that this message has not yet filtered through, even to those who might be thought most likely to hear it (*Health Which?*, 1995). For those who advise the public, the examples of osteopaths and chiropractors in statutory self-regulation are a leap forward. To those other areas in which there are as yet no agreed common standards, we say: get on with it! The absence of a standard safety net is no trivial matter. It is not enough to say, as some have to me, that training or book learning makes no difference to whether somebody is good at healing or not; more training and experience make sound decisions more likely in practice (e.g. in when not to treat, when to refer, recognizing contraindications), and the absence of agreed standards is increasingly likely to undermine consumer confidence in a safe and well-controlled 'transaction'.

For the rest of this chapter I will take a look at Consumers' Association surveys and other data which shed some light on the way in which patients approach complementary therapy, what they have a right to expect from their therapist, and what this means for those offering or regulating therapies.

Who uses complementary therapy, and why

In 1995, a survey of *Which?* members revealed that 31% had used complementary therapy at some time (Table 10.1). Three quarters of those had visited at least one practitioner in the preceding 12 months. This figure of virtually one in four compares with a figure of one in seven in 1986. The people who had used complementary medicine were predominantly women (40% of women were users, versus 27% men); people under 35 were *least* likely to say they had used it (26%, compared to 34% of the 35–64 year olds and 29% of over 65s).

The table also shows the practitioners most commonly visited. Osteopathy, chiropractic and homoeopathy feature strongly, but it may be more surprising to see aromatherapy equal to acupuncture in fourth place. It is clear that people use more than one therapy: in fact 69% of those visiting practitioners in the last 12 months had visited more than one type. It would be tedious to describe the whole complex of interrelated visits, but a couple of examples will suffice. Of the 468 people who had visited a chiropractor, 105 (22%) had also visited an osteopath. That may be to do with the similarity of their therapies in the eyes of patients: both are back workers, and the overlap probably reflects people with back problems shopping around before finding a practitioner they were happy with. However, of the 238 people who

Table 10.1 Consumer responses to 'Have you ever used a practitioner of alternative (complementary) medicine?' (Base = 8745)

Yes	31%
No	65%
No reply	3%
And which of these practitioners have you consulted in the last 12 months? (Base = 2724)	
Osteopath	28%
Chiropractor	17%
Homoeopath	16%
Acupuncturist	12%
Aromatherapist	12%
Reflexologist	9%
Herbalist	6%
Spiritual healer	5%
Hypnotherapist	4%
Alexander teacher	3%
Naturopath	2%
Other practitioner	5%
No visit in last 12 months	23%
No reply	4%

had visited a reflexologist, 93 (39%) had also been to an aromatherapist. Neither of those two therapies is specific enough to say that they are linked by one underlying condition (unless we allow a general term like 'stress-related illness'). Another possible explanation is that these therapies attract people who 'buy in' to the whole approach of complementary medicine – holistic, centred on health (and its promotion) rather than illness (and its cure). We might well conclude that there are two groups of users represented here: those who come with a specific problem to be dealt with, and those who find an approach to life with which they sympathize. Although we must be extremely careful about speculating like this, there is some support for it in the figures.

Table 10.2 looks at the reasons people gave for their last visit to a practitioner. A long-term health problem is the reason most commonly

Table 10.2 Consumer responses to 'What was the reason for your last visit to a practitioner?' (Base = 1874)

New health problem	18%
Long-term health problem	41%
Ongoing consultation/not problem specific	11%
Dissatisfied with orthodox treatment	28%
Because I believe in the general approach of complementary medicine	34%
No reply	13%

given; next is a belief in the general approach; third is dissatisfaction with orthodox treatment. Over half the people who used aromatherapy, spiritual healing, naturopaths and reflexologists gave belief in the general approach as a reason; and women were more likely than men to say this, and significantly more likely than men to be users of aromatherapy. At the same time, osteopathy users were more likely to be men and were more likely to express dissatisfaction with orthodox treatment. So too were users of chiropractic. Chiropractors also (along with spiritual healers) were more likely to be consulted for long-term problems.

The rise of the confident consumer

It would be possible from this to infer not only that there are two types of care, but two types of users of complementary care. There are those, typically men, who use heavy manipulative therapies for tangible, long-term health problems after medics have failed them; the average user of chiropractic or osteopathy clearly comes into this category. Others, likely to be women, use gentler techniques of aromatherapy or reflexology to ease stress, relax and keep them in tune. The implicit sexism of this scenario is only one of its vices; it goes further than the data strictly allow, and the evidence for the divide is circumstantial. But it helps us to think through how a new market in complementary health is growing, as disillusion with orthodox medicine grows. The new market is increasingly made up of people who bring with them real and difficult long-term problems, together with expectations of results and of 'customer service', and they are probably new users. Crudely, men using heavy therapies will fuel the growth of complementary therapy – and they will want results. They are less likely than the traditional patients to buy into the general belief-system of holistic health care. They are less likely to tolerate what *they* regard as unprofessional attitudes (e.g. therapists telling them it will get worse before it gets better). They will have brought their ideas of service from the public sector. Thus they will certainly welcome the extra time they spend with a therapist over a doctor. But, thanks to charters, they are more conscious of a 'right' for treatment to go the way they want it to go.

The role of the under-informed consumer

This new generation of demanding consumers is facing every business in every developed country. They are, in general, better informed and more confident than consumers have ever been before, and have sent big companies scuttling to the customer care consultants to make sure that commerce is ready for them. Complementary therapy should be ready for them, too. But the pundits warn that the new breed of consumers has the potential to act in contradictory ways. In truth they respond differently to different situations. As consumers of health care, and in particular of complementary health care, they are not as well-informed as they ought to be. Neither are they as well-informed as they think they are. The amount of good-quality, objective information available to consumers is low, and its profile is low too.

What is more, consumers have happily carried on consulting practitioners without decent information. Why the willingness to take things on trust? Perhaps it is because of nervousness about health. Perhaps it arises from decades of handing over the responsibility for their good health to white-coated professionals. But whatever the causes, they are more confident of a successful outcome than the evidence will support; over-optimistic about the safety of their treatment; and more confident than they should be of their ability to control the therapist–patient relationship.

Success of therapy

Table 10.3 shows the disparity between how people rate the 'success' of their therapy in tackling the condition they used it for; and (regardless of the outcome) how they feel personally after visiting their practitioner. Thus 46% say therapy has greatly improved their condition, whereas 54% say they feel much better personally after a visit. They are more likely to feel good than the results will technically justify. Table 10.4 shows their satisfaction and the

Table 10.3 Effects of complementary therapies on well-being: consumer responses

Overall, how has the therapy directly affected your condition? (Base = 1874)		*Regardless of the outcome of this therapy, how do you feel after visiting the practitioner? (Base = 1874)*	
Improved greatly	46%	Feel much better	54%
Improved slightly	28%	Feel slightly better	29%
Stayed the same	12%	Feel no different	15%
Deteriorated slightly	1%	Feel slightly worse	1%
Deteriorated greatly	< 1%	Feel much worse	< 1%
Don't know/too soon to say	3%	No reply	< 1%
No pre-existing condition	3%		
No reply	7%		

Table 10.4 Satisfaction with complementary treatment: consumer responses

Taking everything into consideration, how satisfied have you been with your complementary treatment? (Base = 1874)

Very satisfied	54%
Fairly satisfied	30%
Not very satisfied	7%
Not at all satisfied	2%
No reply	7%

numbers are very closely related to how they feel after a visit (e.g. 54% very satisfied).

Notice, incidentally, how puzzlingly few cite 'no pre-existing condition' – just 3%. In Table 10.2, by contrast, 11% said their reason for treatment was 'part of an ongoing series of consultations, or not problem-specific'. The disparity may be accounted for by the people who did not answer, or by differences in the questions. Or it may be by the human instinct towards contradictory behaviour: they may *say* they do not want to measure success by anything so crude as concrete results to a health problem, but a yardstick of problem-solving seems to be in their minds when they are asked to judge.

Over-optimistic on safety of treatment

It is important to stress to even fairly sophisticated consumers that what is often called natural medicine is not necessarily safe medicine, and that the physiological effects of injections, acupuncture, X-rays, manipulation or herbal medicines are not always negligible. Data from Professor Ernst (see Chapter 8) suggest that consumers under-estimate the risk of side effects. When asked why they used complementary medicine, 48% said they wanted a cure without side effects (while 32% expressed themselves disappointed with orthodox medicine). If only this were true of all complementary medicine! It may be that side effects are a real risk but comparatively rare: a review in *Acupuncture in Medicine* (1995) concluded that there had been 216 reports in the journals of complications arising from acupuncture over the last 20 years. Even a small number is unacceptable, however. A woman reported in *Health Which?* (1985) that her osteopath had punctured a lung by injecting her incompetently. From the patient's point of view, how many punctured lungs are acceptable?

Complaints systems are not used

In a *Health Which?* survey of dissatisfied consumers of complementary medicine, we found a low rate of people wishing to complain: 85 out of 2635, or 3%. We interviewed 33 people in depth, and found that barely any had consulted a register before choosing a practitioner. After their visit, only two went on to make a formal complaint. One used a solicitor, who looked up registration details for her. She was the only one to receive compensation. In all, three people contacted a professional body direct: two found that their practitioner was not a member, and a third had no reply to her letter. In preparation for the same article, the British Complementary Medicine Association told us they have received no complaints about their members. But our research suggests that this is very different from saying that nobody has a complaint. People (and *Health Which?* subscribers ought to be the best informed people of all) simply do not know where to go for a reliable practitioner, nor where to turn if they have a complaint. There is much profile-raising to be done before the consumer of complementary medicine is able to make an informed choice with a decent chance of redress if things go wrong.

The temptation to do nothing

It would of course be possible to continue to take advantage of this situation of under-informed consumers for as long as it lasts. Tempting, too. After all, belief is an important ingredient in healing, and explaining the limitations of treatment may undermine that belief and thereby harm success rates – even against the interest of the individual patient. It may put people off treatment altogether to explain to them that, for example, aromatherapy massage has not been proved to relieve lower back pain. After all, the lack of randomized controlled trial evidence does not mean it will not do that particular person some good. Besides, the present goodwill towards complementary medicine, whereby 79% would recommend it to a friend, is based on positive experience, not on written evidence. Word of mouth and instinct are important factors in choice. Why rock the boat?

Enlightening under-informed consumers

Despite the convenience of under-informed consumers, it is imperative that we should disabuse the innocent consumers of any unreasoning faith in complementary therapies. Their very evident present satisfaction is unlikely to be undermined by good honest information, and there are real dangers ahead if consumers stay under-informed. There are two parallel sets of arguments: the ethical (comprising safety and efficacy) and the self-interested.

Safety

Take the ethical case first, and look at safety. In a consumer society, we very often enumerate consumer principles of rights to access, choice, information, redress and safety. The greatest of these is safety. The consumer movement will support interference in a free market, or over-ride unlimited choice when safety is at stake. We do not, therefore, argue that your local butcher should be free to give you chiropractic treatment. Patients in any sort of health care deserve safe treatment; if this cannot be guaranteed, they deserve to know about the risks they run. They also have the right to a level of competence which determines when to refer to a medical practitioner; when treatment should be stopped. They also deserve protection against abuse, physical or mental, and it is absolutely necessary for more whistleblowers in complementary medicine, to isolate and drive out the bad guys. The avenues for complaint and redress offered to the tiny minority of disappointed customers need to be wider and better signposted; practically nobody uses them at the moment, and that is not because nobody has any complaints.

Efficacy

Ethically again, we must expect to offer to patients only health care treatments where there is a reasonable chance of success. This is true of any therapy, orthodox or complementary, and it means that we are obliged to collect and give to patients trustworthy and relevant evidence. Consumers should be able to predict that the effects of their treatment will be better than no treatment, or than the unsuccessful treatment they had before. Without such evidence, only the practitioner's experience and judgment can predict the likely outcome. And as doctors have been finding to their cost, the interference of individual hunches and personal beliefs in a given treatment mean that subjective judgments are not enough. The concept of evidence-based medicine arose to solve just that problem.

We have seen how disillusionment with orthodox medicine appears to be feeding the growth of complementary medicine. Some commentators have suggested that people have simply transferred their faith in doctors to complementary practitioners. There is the concomitant risk that some of them will follow on by transferring their disillusionment. If anything, complementary therapy needs to outstrip orthodox medicine in putting the patient first: not only because it is so reliant on private fees, but because of the holistic principles which almost all therapies espouse. It would be ironic if practitioners who put patients at the centre of their healing practice fail to make people the centre of their professional values.

As with safety arguments, so with efficacy: the only ethical course is to gather information and to share it. At the moment, a consumer's choice is based on factors like word of mouth and media reports, but they deserve to be able to make an informed choice based on scientific information. It is unacceptable to exploit the patient's lack of knowledge to allow treatment to carry on without the backing of evidence or consideration of risk. You cannot ethically take advantage of the under-informed consumer for the sake of an easy life.

Therapists' own interest in spreading information

It is not all gloom. The interests of complementary therapy in general sit well with the ethical case for more information. Getting informed consent puts the practitioner in a stronger position if there should be any complaint. Gathering evidence of efficacy and following it in clinical practice also helps in defence, should any practitioner, heaven forbid, be the subject of a complaint or litigation. Sharing information means that your patients have more realistic expectations, and less likelihood of disappointment. Better handling of complaints, as all businesses have found, leads to more repeat custom. In fact, some customer care research indicates that a customer whose complaint has been well-handled is more likely to be a repeat customer than somebody who never complained! With a professionally run system of complaints handling, disappointment can be minimized, and cause for complaint acknowledged and dealt with, before the consequences become too bitter. To carry on with a poor or low profile system risks a pool of unvoiced complaints, which could at some future time turn into a poisonous flood of media scares or public ill-will. The interests of complementary therapy lie in running tight systems of self-regulation which are responsive to patients' needs and wishes. The alternative is compulsory regulation imposed from outside.

The implications for registration

A patient may be bemused to find that there are half a dozen or more bodies that his or her reflexologist might belong to or have trained with. An author or a health professional recommending (for example) the Society of Teachers of the Alexander Technique may be taken aback by the offence caused to other membership organizations which subsequently protest that they have not been included. But it is not an outsider's place to bring therapists together, or to offer a solution to the maze of different therapy organizations. That must be the job of mature professional therapists coming to agreement among themselves. If the complementary sector desires respect and trust among the public at large, it must deserve it. And sorting out the internecine rivalries between groups representing the same therapy must be the most important step towards a professional outlook.

Conclusion

Patients are as a rule not interested in the politics of their therapy. They are primarily interested in getting well. Patients are less concerned than therapists about small points of difference between registration bodies over registration, different modes of evaluation, and different types of training. There are many reasons for this. It is not an outsider's business; a patient trusts in anybody they perceive as a health professional; the matters of disagreement between therapists and doctors (or between therapists and therapists!) are a long way from the concerns of the patient or potential patient.

So the future for complementary therapy is to rally the cause of the under-informed consumer. For the complementary therapy profession, this means:

- a commitment to informed consent, recognizing the implications for the efficacy of treatment, which will not always be to the benefit of the patient or help the therapy
- practice information: giving out reliable, professional information about the suitability of treatment for various conditions, likelihood of success, and details of relevant registration bodies. These could be brought together in something like a practice leaflet. A commitment to rigorous evaluation by trials is implicit in giving out information
- publicizing the role of the professional and registering bodies more widely, and helping people to complain or to blow the whistle on unacceptable practice or practitioners. Paradoxically, this is likely to improve the loyalty of clients and improve the image of complementary therapy, as well as meeting growing public expectation from confident consumers about their rights.

It is up to practitioners in complementary medicine to see that any misapprehensions of consumers are put right. Above all, if disillusion is not to set in here as it has in orthodox healthcare, the lessons of sharing information with consumers must be learned and acted upon.

References

Rampes, H. and James, R. (1995) Complications of acupuncture. *Acupuncture in Medicine*, May. p. 26

Anon for *Health Which?* (1995) Risking the alternatives. *Health Which?*, December. p. 196

Anon for *Which?* (1986) Complementary medicine. *Which?*, October. p. 443

Anon for *Which?* (1995) Healthy choice. *Which?*, November. p. 8

Index